AF413694

STORIES
OF OUR
LIVES

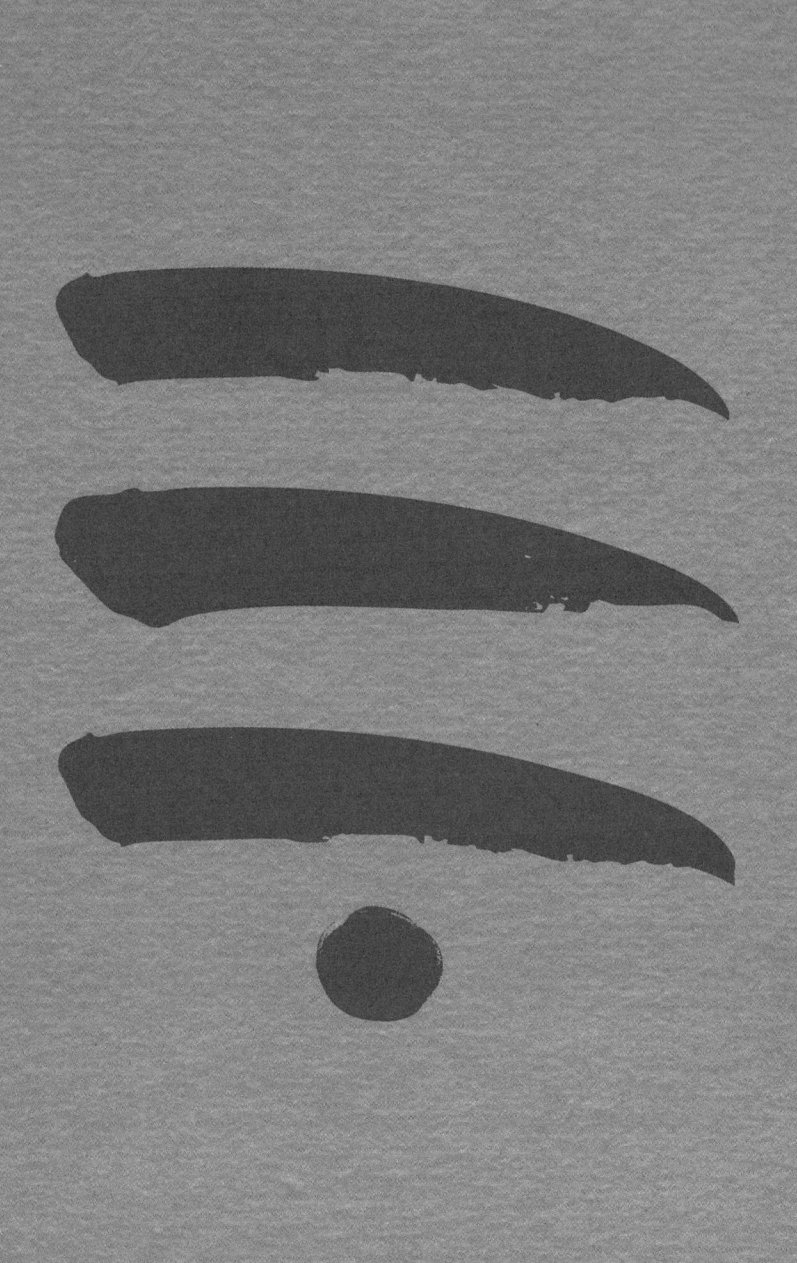

STORIES OF OUR LIVES

OF OUR LIVES

AWAKENED LIVING THROUGH SACRED MYTHOLOGY

JANET STONE

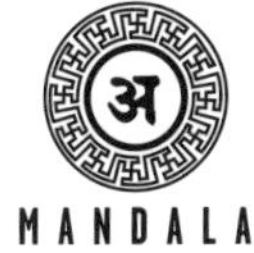

MANDALA

San Rafael Los Angeles London

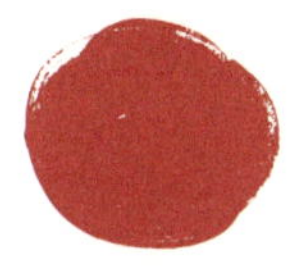

CONTENTS

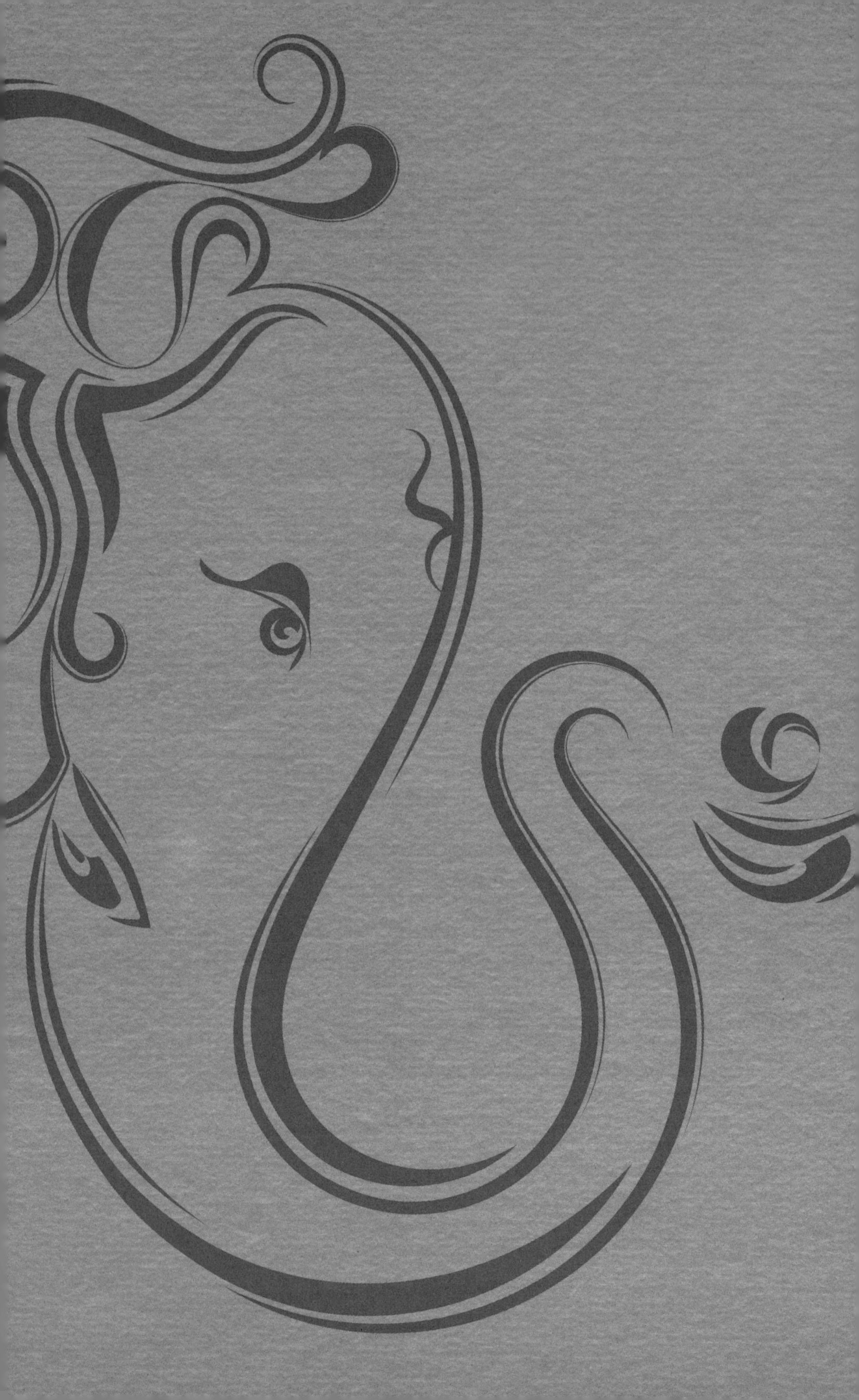

●

AND SO IT BEGINS . . .

Stories are a communal currency of humanity.

—Tahir Shah, *In Arabian Nights*

Kali was coming to my house.

It was New Year's Eve. I was twenty-one years old and should have been out partying. Instead, I crawled into the hospital bed set up for my father in our living room while his brain cancer metastasized. He had slipped into a coma that morning. His body was limp, his eyes closed, and as I wrapped my arm around him, I placed my lips close to his face and whispered the unthinkable in his ear: that it was okay for him to go, to let go of his body, to die. Not one part of me wanted to say these words, but I knew how important it was to let him know that he could go, that I would be okay, that I would take care of Mom and live a life he would be proud of. I listened closely to the labor of his breath and sobbed quietly on his slack shoulder.

After a fitful sleep that night, my body sprung awake when I heard my mom's small voice call down to my bedroom. At my father's bedside in minutes, I joined my mom, my sister, and my grandmother. As he labored for each breath, we held him and talked to him, repeating "I love you" over and over.

Kali was here.

At 8:05 a.m. on that New Year's morning, my father's breath slowed to a near imperceptible inhale, followed by an extended exhale. My hand over his heart, I waited with every bit of hope, wishing, willing, and pleading for the next breath to arrive. After many minutes that felt like days and months waiting for the next breath, it struck me that it was never coming again. That was his last breath. As his strong, young body lay there, his skin still warm under my hand, I could see, plain as day, that his essence had left his body.

Kali, the goddess of destruction, with blood dripping from her outstretched tongue, eyes rolled back in her head, a necklace of skulls cascading around her dark-blue shimmering neck, and her wild tangle of hair like fire burning in the black night sky, had come and taken my father, leaving in her wake an unnamable void, seemingly unending grief, and a deep search for meaning.

After my father's death, I came across a story of goddess Kali in a college book and felt assured by this radical figure who gives by taking. I had never before heard of Kali, but suddenly I was fascinated. To my understanding, her gift was destruction. She comes for everything we hold sacred, every single thing we hold on to—including our family, our nearest and dearest, our stories, our certainties, and, eventually, our bodies.

In her destruction, she offers the grace of infinite formlessness, the vast eternal. In the story of Kali, I experienced an odd sense of familiarity and what I might call relief or feeling understood. In her timeless story, I immersed myself in a mythology that showed me another way of seeing the coming and going of souls.

And so it begins . . .

STORIES: THE THREADS OF HUMAN EXISTENCE

Stories are the threads in the fabric of human existence, the universal language that transcends time and culture. We need stories to understand ourselves. We need stories to understand the world. Stories invite us to remember a deeper nature that tends to get lost in our daily dramas. They are a way of seeing ourselves and the human condition through a boundless lens, a view from the stars. They invite our connection with the eternal flow of life. It's as if we can peek behind the current of our personal narrative and unveil the richness that interconnects all living things.

Stories have the power to evoke tears, passion, and wonder, to set us out on new adventures, to bring us closer, and to tear us apart. Stories are the great wisdom keepers, joy makers, sorrow trackers, and inspiration to so many. Whether told orally, as they have been traditionally, or in writing, they can stir up lost parts within us. To immerse ourselves in an ancient story is to remember parts of ourselves we may have long forgotten. The great legends bridge our mundane existence with cosmic phenomena, aligning the heartbeat of humanity with the rhythm of the universe.

The stories I am about to share with you are puranas—ancient tales from India. These legends are woven from a collective understanding of the nature of the mind, body, and spirit, offering a road map back to our inherent oneness and the many faces of our life's experience.

MY JOURNEY WITH THE PURANAS

Before we begin, let's first confront the obvious: I'm not from India. I'm a California girl, living, learning, and sharing these stories. So why am I so entranced by the puranas? These stories guided me in my darkest hours, inspired me in moments I felt lost, and became a beacon through the ups and downs of life, love, and death. But how did these stories reach me, living all the way on the other side of the planet?

I attribute this to my grandfather, his parents, and my great-great-grandfather. You see, three generations of my family were born and raised in India. As a family of doctors and missionaries on the outskirts of Hyderabad, my ancestors spent their lives with the local farmers and laborers. They were surrounded by India, its beliefs, and its rich art of storytelling. From what I'm told, the local stories wove into the Western beliefs of my grandfather and his siblings. From the way they lived, my younger self could sense that something about them was different from other families. Through my great-grand-mother, great-aunt, and grandfather, the essence of these fables made it to me and awakened an entirely unique world within.

To put it simply, these puranas have molded and changed my life in countless ways. Hearing them opened new worlds, each imbued with wisdom, morals, and perspectives that challenged and stretched my understanding of life and reality.

Throughout my life's twists and turns, I have found myself sharing the puranas across the globe, from corporate events at Google, where I recounted Hanuman's leap—with the message that being reminded of our inherent superpowers by those around us can help us to fly—to a yoga festival in Beijing, where I shared the story of Krishna and Radha's unity and devotion to love. I've referred countless yoga students to the myriad books, texts, and teachers that have inspired me and given me an understanding of the power of puranas.

These stories aren't mine; they are told in endless variations and infinite versions, in an ever-changing flow of wisdom that feeds those who hear them with exactly what they may need to receive in the moment.

MY STORY

As a child, the story I lived was that of a Northern Californian, quasi-hippie family, living off the land, milking goats, carting wool, and rescuing any and all orphaned animals. We raised boa constrictors, raccoons, opossums, birds, deer, koi, squirrels— whatever needed help, we rescued it.

Right alongside modern Americana, my family ran around half naked or in handmade clothes, churning butter and making nature our playground, while our contemporaries took tennis lessons and ate bologna on white bread. Sometimes I felt like an outcast, as if I had been dropped into the wrong story, as if I was somehow not in the right time or the right place, like I was an outsider in my own neighborhood.

While other families gathered around the TV at night, we didn't have one and would instead tell stories and make up epic sagas with our animals as characters, feeding a rich imagination. Growing up in the creeks, fields, and trees, riding bareback on horses, and being surrounded by so many animals peeled open my imagination and unconsciously set me on my lifelong journey to seek a deeper truth—one that felt accessible through these old tales and through my relationship with nature.

On this journey I faced my own dramas. The traumatic deaths of many loved ones led me to a search for meaning and taught me from a young age that this life is temporary. Everything is impermanent. From human to animal life, it was all coming and going. What was it all for? What was it all about?

My teachers of impermanence included our adorable, fluffy bunnies, our clucky, sweet chickens, and our bouncy goats and sheep. It was my chore to take care of them, and I would fall in love with each and every one of them only to learn that some of them would be butchered, and I had to help in that process. I went from loving and tending them to seeing my bunnies hanging by the back foot tendon while I was taught to gut and skin them, later finding it on my dinner plate. The journey from being alive in my arms to being on the dinner table was a potent lesson in life's impermanence, to say the least.

At seventeen I was living in Boulder, Colorado, attending high school. On weekends and school breaks, I traveled with a professional cover band, singing backup, dancing, and playing the tambourine. At one of our events in Aspen, I expressed my search for greater understanding of life's mysteries to the lead singer, who promptly introduced me to the teachings of Maharaji. I eventually became a student and aspirant of his teachings. This is when the door of meditation opened for me. With meditation as my grounding force, no matter where I went, I could find my way home.

Later I worked for Castle Rock Entertainment during the *Seinfeld* era, in an office with the likes of Billy Crystal, Larry David (the cocreator of *Seinfeld*), Rob Reiner, Alan Zweibel, and other amazing writers, directors, and producers. Starting as a production assistant, I eventually made my own short films, and even wrote a sitcom pilot, though it didn't end up being produced.

THE CALL TO ADVENTURE

Many years into my LA life and film-industry career, I found myself at the premiere of a movie in Beverly Hills, surrounded by the likes of Michael Douglas, Annette Bening, and Rob Reiner. Amid the noise I felt a flood of calm wash over me. I'd recently had an abortion and found myself in a deep well of despair and grief. But, in that moment my heart rate slowed, my feet were grounded, and I stood holding a plate of hors d'oeuvres, which included rabbit satay, while the famous made small talk. In that moment everything faded around me and I heard a call from within—a call that urged me to run toward the great unknown of the world, a call that would have me abandon this life in Hollywood I'd worked so hard to create.

It was the call of the hero's journey.

When I'd moved to LA I took film classes at UCLA, and my very first class was on screenwriting. We read Joseph Campbell's *The Hero with a Thousand Faces*. Campbell referred to the Bhagavad Gita and other ancient texts and mythologies as he broke down the arc of a great myth. This helped me see how every story had a unifying structure. This was my first introduction to the Gita and its rich epic of Krishna and Arjuna and the inevitable battle Arjuna faces—the one we must all face. These story arcs, once seen clearly, showed up for me in every script, book, or movie that I saw or read afterward.

Campbell lays out how in *The Hero's Journey*, we meet the hero in their ordinary world, witnessing some moment that forces them out of this comfort and into what Campbell calls "the adventure." Then comes the resistance to this call, meeting a mentor along the way, the crossing of some threshold and being unable to turn back, the meetings of enemies and allies, enduring tests, then arriving at the innermost cave, the ordeal that unfolds, the reward for the battle faced, the road back, resurrection, and the final return to the ordinary yet forever changed.

I was standing there at the premiere, feeling an indescribable pull to step toward the unknown. This moment is what I recognized as the call of the heart, the call that Joseph Campbell speaks of, the call to break out of my comfort zone and go on my adventure. The study of *The Hero's Journey* gave me insight that following the call wouldn't be easy, but it would be a worthy adventure and would bring me back to myself. But would I answer it?

I loved what I did. I loved the film industry. It was my ideal life of creativity, learning, community, growth, and I even found a way to thrive in the beauty and nature of Los Angeles through surfing, mountain biking, skydiving, ocean swimming, and trail running. I was living a life I couldn't have even dreamed of. I had everything, and yet, in the quiet of the chaos around me at the premiere, I knew I had to listen to this inner call.

So I took the first step on *my* hero's journey. I sold my belongings, let go of my oceanfront apartment, packed up my life in LA, and headed on a solo journey around the world with my mountain bike, snowboard, and one backpack. Through Egypt, Europe, India, Nepal, Cambodia, Laos, Vietnam, Thailand, Indonesia, Australia, New Zealand, Fiji, and so on, I journeyed.

My time, particularly in India, only fed my hunger to study and understand the puranas more deeply. While on this search in the Tamil Nadu region of India, I came across the teachings of Ramana Maharshi, an Indian Hindu sage who died in 1950, leaving behind a legacy of teachings that asked the big questions: Who am I? Who is the narrator of my story?

It was the message I needed at the time. This was my mentor or guide in the sequence of my hero's journey. Along the way I met a lot of challenges and setbacks but kept enduring along the path. Ramana's teachings not only encouraged me to sit with the why, but also enlightened me about the illusion of the who; to essentially look behind the curtain like our dear Dorothy does in *The Wizard of Oz*. They taught me that the one asking the question and the one answering it are not separate. They are but the reflections of the same consciousness experiencing itself.

After my journey around the world, where I'd picked up the multifaceted yoga practices including the movement yoga we know so well today, I returned to LA and continued studying yoga in the mid- to late '90s and early 2000s. I also returned to the film industry, working on HBO's *Curb Your Enthusiasm*, created by Larry David.

I had finally returned back from my adventure, back to my ordinary life, yet I was forever changed.

LIVING THE PURANAS

In between film projects, yoga began to take on a larger role in my life, and I found myself teaching it to film-industry friends, to surfer friends at the beach, and to anyone and everyone who would join me. Soon I found myself teaching yoga more than working on industry projects, and the stories and chanting (the invocation of the deity energy through song) became some of the ways I shared this tradition.

This shift from filmmaking to teaching yoga felt like a natural progression, intertwining my love for storytelling with the ancient wisdom of the puranas, and creating a unique blend of physical movement, myth, and meditation. I found that the stories resonated deeply with my students, just as they had with me. The more I shared, the more I felt called to delve into these myths and bring their timeless wisdom to a broader audience.

So here I am, a woman born in California, called to share these stories from a time and place that are not mine. This is a testament to the universality of these stories. They transcend geographical boundaries and cultural divides, reaching out to anyone who is willing to listen, learn, understand, and be moved by them.

I am acutely aware of the thousands of years these stories have been passed down, the meaning they carry for so many, and the privilege of hearing and sharing them through chanting and retelling. The process of writing them down comes after much deep dialogue with my teachers in India, each one encouraging me to share the stories as far and widely as possible so that they may live on.

The stories are finally put onto these pages after decades of telling and retelling, with each iteration taking on a life of its own, and each listener hearing the part of the story that resonates with them. The stories meet us at the moment we're in and guide us to know ourselves and the many aspects of ourselves more intimately.

Every line in this book, every anecdote shared, every character and plot twist, is imbued with the hope that as you journey through these pages, you too will experience the life-changing power of these timeless narratives and make them a part of your own story.

A GAME OF TELEPHONE

To give you some context, there are eighteen major (*mukhya*) and eighteen minor (*upa*) puranas, encompassing approximately four hundred thousand verses. They are not considered scriptures like the Vedas, but are called smritis, which translates to "reminiscences" or "memories." This is helpful to me in understanding and working with puranas, in that we are individually and collectively remembering some aspects of ourselves that may have been buried.

Most scholars regard these myths as the work of numerous unknown authors over centuries, continually expanded, edited, and reshaped in their evolution—like an endless game of telephone. The stories morph and shift with each speaker and each listener. They are still a work in process, right up to this very moment as you read the stories on these pages. Through these ancient Hindu puranas, we unearth the profound cellular truth that connects us all and binds us in the human story—a living story.

In Western thought, we often value information and shun myths as irrational, childish, or unreasonable. Most of what we applaud as important is data—disjointed bits and pieces of information devoid of the infinite story of life, rather than living and breathing wisdom. Somewhere along the way we've lost the connection to what lies deep within our cells, our intuition, and mystical inner design.

The puranas are meant to awaken the patterns and complexity of our wondrous innate wisdom. What I'm sharing here is neither scholastic nor text-driven; these are the interpretations of my feeling, breathing, living experience of these great stories.

OUR STORY

None of us can pinpoint exactly where we are in the plot of our lives. This uncertainty can be both terrifying and liberating. All too often we assume we have a certain amount of time based on certain expectations, and we go about tossing precious moments away, lost in the swirl of dramas, confusion, and misperceptions.

When we hear a story that resonates with our experience and reveals aspects of ourselves we have yet to fully perceive, it allows us to see ourselves and the world around us more fully. Through these stories, my hope is that we can step outside ourselves and look back with clear eyes. The number of times I get lost in misperception is incalculable, and the guidance of these stories to provide me with context and a clearer seeing has been my journey to widen my perspective.

Here's one such instance: In the mid-'90s I was in Kathmandu. I had been dreaming of trekking to Everest Base Camp for years, and finally, after many months in Egypt and India, with a myriad of thresholds, each one putting my will to persevere to a more severe test than the last, I had finally landed in Kathmandu to prepare for my trek. Along with my snowboard and climbing gear, I brought a crumpled copy of the Indian epic the Ramayana that I'd picked up at some gloomy $1.30-a-night hostel in India, which I read voraciously.

The anticipation was high as I met with my trek guides and settled on the final details of the itinerary. With some time to explore Kathmandu, I headed to Swayambhunath Temple with my camera and curiosity—solo travel allows for so much time to wander. There, I spun the giant prayer wheels and found precociously adorable monkeys to photograph. Engrossed in capturing their play, I failed to notice the agitated mama monkey until I suddenly felt a jolt of weight on my back and a sharp burning sensation as her fangs dug into my flesh. With shock and confusion, I began screaming and flailing around. Finally, satisfied that I'd learned my lesson and that her baby was safe, she leapt off, leaving the bystanders perhaps more stunned than I was.

Feeling the warmth of blood dripping down my back, I made my way to the international medical clinic. As I sat in the waiting room, hurried staff rushed outside to meet an incoming ambulance and rushed in two men with extreme cases of frostbite. I later learned that they were the men rescued on Everest after their guide and three other climbers died on the mountain. Suddenly my monkey bite seemed insignificant. I was finally treated and told that I would either have to delay my trek or self-administer rabies shots for several weeks. I chose the latter.

I packed up my needles and serum and headed to the Tenzing-Hillary Airport in Lukla, the tiny mountain village that hosts one of the highest airports on the planet, to begin my journey toward Base Camp. As I boarded the ten-seater airplane, I remembered the part in the Ramayana where

Hanuman heads to the Himalayas. He was tasked with saving Lakshmana's life and had to procure a life-saving herb from the Himalayas. However, when he got there, he couldn't identify the correct herb, so he grabbed the entire mountain. Here I was bringing a canister of serum to the Himalayas, yet I could feel the strength and determination of Hanuman in my pursuit. This whole journey around the world was my longing to heal from my father's death, from recent heartbreak, an abortion, grief and internal confusion, to come closer to the truth of life, and Hanuman's unwavering resolve reminded me that no matter how lost or insignificant I might feel, I possess the power to overcome obstacles and find my way. His story became my source of inspiration, guiding me through and helping me realize that the answers I sought were within me all along.

In the face of all the stories I've lived through, the puranas have helped take me beyond the surface of this character of I/me/mine, into the fabric of *being*—the forces that propel me along this path. They beg the question: Can we still hold the thread of ancient wisdom and yet weave something new?

In the Indian pantheon of gods and goddesses, the One is expressed through many, or the many express the One. It creates a home for all of us—we are a divine form; we are a demon; we are a goddess who has lost her cool or a god who has fallen prey to egoic pursuits; we are a wild, untethered fierceness slaying all attachment. We are an ever-changing expression of the One.

Within these pages, when I refer to the ego or the I/me/mine structure, it is not with a negative connotation. It is to express the Hindu concept of *ahamkara*—how the soul (*atman*) associates with the physical body. In everyday language, *ahamkara* means "arrogance" or "pride," but in the broader sense it is the separation of the self from the rest of the creation and the Creator.

Ahamkara is derived from the Sanskrit words *aham* (meaning "I") and *kara* (meaning "maker" or "doer"), literally translating to "the making of the I." It is the principle that gives rise to the ego, the sense of individual identity that makes us perceive ourselves as distinct entities separate from the rest of the universe. This sense of individuality is necessary for navigating the physical world, allowing us to differentiate between ourselves and others, to make decisions, and to build our lives. However, when the ego becomes overly dominant, it leads to a distorted sense of self, characterized by excessive pride, arrogance, and attachment to material possessions and personal achievements.

In the context of the puranas, we can see *ahamkara* as a double-edged sword. On one hand it is a vital aspect of our existence; on the other hand it is a source of suffering, creating a false sense of separation from the divine and the interconnected web of life. The puranas invite us to recognize this dual nature of *ahamkara* and to cultivate a balanced relationship with it. It's not about annihilating the ego but rather about integrating it into a broader, more expansive understanding of the self. By softening our grip on our ego, we can transcend the illusion of separateness and experience oneness with the divine—a great level of peace and freedom from suffering. Even in a moment of great pain and fear, bleeding from the bite of a literal monkey on our back, we can recognize that our suffering is not the only suffering in the world. We are bound to others, who may be suffering even greater pain and loss than we are, and we can draw courage and even healing to move forward with our journey from that sense of shared experience.

THE POWER OF CURIOSITY

The puranas are stories that are not only for entertainment; they offer new ways to understand ourselves and the universal themes that play into our lives, bringing the collective unconscious to life. They can also build a stronger personal practice and awareness of internal guiding forces. To see ourselves as the heroes or as the shadow characters in a story allows us to gain perspective on our own selves and all the many characters we play in this lifetime or even in a given day. The puranas reveal the masks we put on in order to fit in, to manage, or to seemingly trick ourselves and those around us. However, living a life with a false persona only causes suffering. The puranas invite us on the heroic path of digging within to reveal our many faces and give ourselves the bountiful gift of integrating and expressing all aspects of ourselves.

When we begin to look at ourselves through the lens of the puranas and the archetypes they portray, it's like a play in which we're acting out love and loss, likes and dislikes, and fears and confidence. In this grand cosmic play, *you* are a vital character too. You are the hero, the villain, the sage, the fool—a multifaceted being, capable of infinite growth and transformation.

As we set foot into the expansive world of the puranas, let us remember to bring along our most essential tool: curiosity. For it is through curiosity that we begin to see beyond the surface and into the heart of these eternal stories.

The power of the sacred resides among us. Are we willing to tune in? Are we willing to listen, look, and feel our way into these narratives to allow them to transform us? These stories pause the relentless flow of the mundane and immerse us in sacred wisdom, a deeper knowing and understanding, opening the door to the potential of waking up.

SACRED LISTENING

Sravana is the ancient art and joy of listening to divine stories and bathing in their symbology. Here we will do just that—immerse ourselves in ancient stories that echo our modern experiences. The richness of wisdom, spiritual teachings, and epic stories was traditionally passed down through oral recitation. Even though I am sharing the stories with you in written form, I believe we can open the inner aperture of our ears to listen to the deep understanding sparked by the tale. The art of truly hearing stories brings us more intimately face-to-face with our own subconscious. It allows us to suspend sureness and drift into the realm of remembering that our stories are a powerful thread—born of a specific time and place but capturing universal themes of the human experience. While we're alive, we simply get to hold onto this thread, and if we're curious enough to step back from our daily dramas, we will see how this thread is woven through time, connecting us to all who came before us and all who will come after us.

We live in a modern world where information comes our way faster than we can comprehend, discern, or feel. Our ears have tuned into false narratives that lead us down paths that have us believing in the illusion of social media, and messages of division, fear, outrage, and that somehow we're not enough. When we share the stories of the great universal struggle of light versus shadow, we are able to see that even the most revered beings struggle with their inner forces. This is the reinforcement we need to lift ourselves out of the collective *maya* (illusion) that we can get so lost in. In the chaos of information that floods our world, listening to these stories offers us a beacon of clarity, guiding us through the *maya* and reminding us of our common origins and shared destiny.

SACRED SEEING

Darshan is the ancient practice of auspiciously seeing (in form or in one's own mind's eye) a deity, a guru (teacher), or something that brings illumination. While hearing the tales of the gods and goddesses, we can use the sense of sight to look inward and to see these deities within us as well as in the world around us. We can also look at a picture or a *murti* (sacred statue), nature, or anything else that may inspire a deeper connection with the essence of the myth.

Our perspective shapes our understanding, and if we broaden our perspective, like a camera panning back, we can take in the infinite tapestry of life—not only human life, but *all* life and its divine interconnectedness. How can we look at another person, being, or group of people and determine that we are better or worse, when we all make up this same tapestry? These old patterns of seeing keep us stuck on a roller coaster, unable to look with curiosity at the world around us. They keep us wandering through our days on the yo-yo of self-loathing and self-aggrandizement. Our work is to open our eyes and begin to see the divine within and all around.

SACRED FEELING

Bhava—the feelings, emotions, or vibe of an experience—is a core aspect of stories. The realm of *bhava* is where we truly connect with the heart of the stories. When we embrace the feeling state of the puranas, we engage with the *navarasas*, the nine emotions: *shringara* (love or beauty), *hasya* (laughter), *karuna* (sorrow), *rudra* (anger), *vira* (heroism or courage), *bhayanaka* (terror or fear), *bibhatsa* (disgust), *adbutha* (surprise or wonder), and *shantha* (peace or tranquility). Embracing the *navarasas* allows us to deeply engage with these tales while also exploring our own emotional landscape.

All of these emotions give us permission to be *feeling* beings in the world. The power of a story to invoke the many feeling states of human experience can give us a better understanding of our own subconscious push and pull. When we allow the feelings to flow, we allow ourselves to drop behind the frontal lobe—the part of the brain's cerebrum that is responsible for our thought processes—and access the occipital cortex or the temporal lobe—the parts of the brain that process senses and feeling. Through a story, we enter the realms of intuition and emotion rather than being stuck in the cognitive realm of thinking.

Our journey through the oral tradition is not just about *sravana*, *darshan*, or *bhava*—listening, seeing, or feeling; it's a dynamic interplay of all three. We become active participants in these timeless tales, breathing life into them, and in the process, discovering a deeper understanding of ourselves and our place in the grand tapestry of life.

This list of the feelings, experiences, and expressions captures elements of ourselves and aspects of our shared humanity. Each one has a story to tell, a lesson of humans longing for meaning, purpose, and connection—truly an intense longing for remembering.

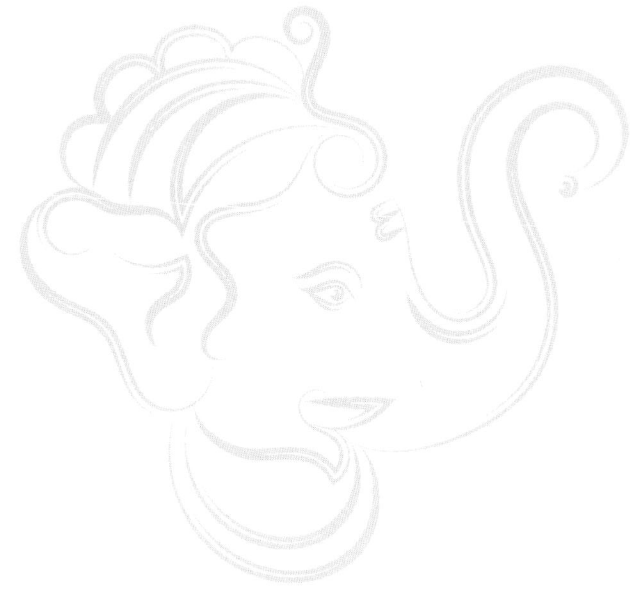

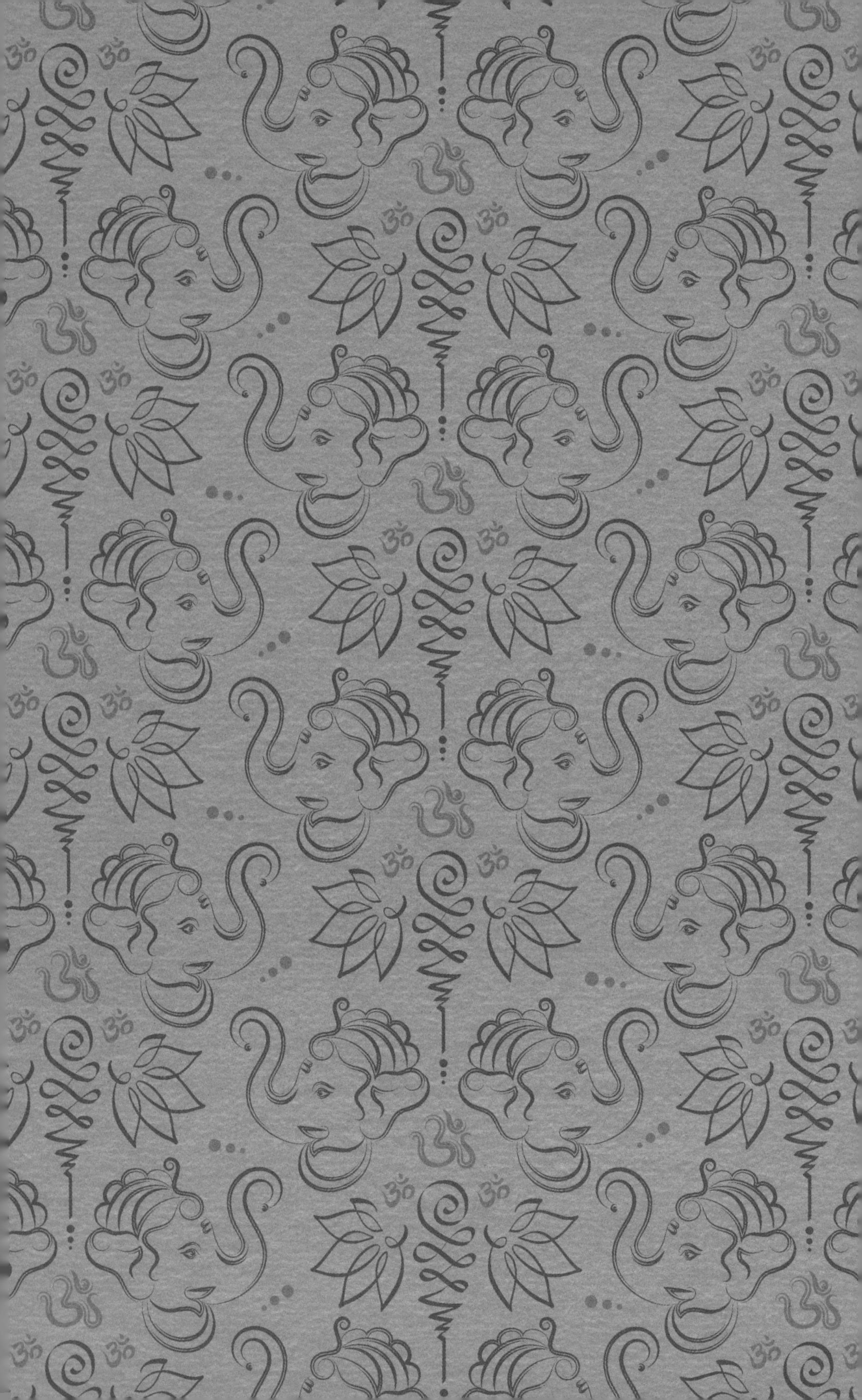

ROAD MAP TO THIS BOOK

Each chapter in this book focuses on a different purana and is divided into three sections. In the first section, I tell you the story—a good old-fashioned tale, a place to lose oneself. Here, we drop behind the analytical mind and float in the spaces in between, allowing the sweet nectar to drip, drip, drip into the mind, body, and soul. This first section allows our intuition to remember that we are all of the characters in all of these stories.

The second section, "Myth and Meaning," is a light, secular exploration of the puranic tale that allows us to reengage our frontal lobe—the analytical mind—and make sense of the feelings and emotions of the story. This section is about creating space for integration and insight into our own lives, feelings, and stories.

The final section in each chapter, "Myth into Practice," explores ways to practice and incorporate the purana's wisdom into our daily lives. As a practitioner of meditation and the art and science of yoga for over thirty years, I can say without a doubt that without practice we revert to old behaviors, patterns, and loops. And as my friend and teacher Hareesh Wallis would say, "knowledge without practice is a burden."

The practices in this book are designed to facilitate that experience and help integrate it into our mental constructs and our very cells. In each "Myth into Practice" section you'll find the below elements to help you incorporate the teaching in your life.

MANTRA: This means "mind tool" in Sanskrit, the language of the Vedas and Yoga Sutras, and in the oral traditions of yoga before these early texts. It's often a repetition of words (in Sanskrit or your primary language) that helps you return to center and invoke an intention. These mantras can be chanted or spoken and are used to pull your mind back toward your intended desire to invoke or bring about the energy of the deity/character in the story told. Most mantras are repeated 108 times; however, if you're just starting out, you can repeat them nine times. I recommend consistently returning to these mantras and simply noting any internal or external changes in your life.

MEDITATION: These are written guided contemplative exercises. Since they are written, you have to open your eyes at moments to read the text. You can read the meditation prompts and pause afterward for five to twenty-four minutes to allow yourself to experience the guidance.

MOVEMENT: If you have a yoga asana practice (or any kind of movement practice), I invite you to explore these themes in your body. If you have physical limitations, these practices can encompass just the movement you're able to access, whether it's with the eyes, the upper torso, the limbs, or the whole body.

EXERCISES: These are experiential actions that you can explore as you go about your day or week. Most are designed to be explorations within very common daily experiences, such as a conversation or a journal entry. Use your current journal, if you have one, or pick one up to use just with this book.

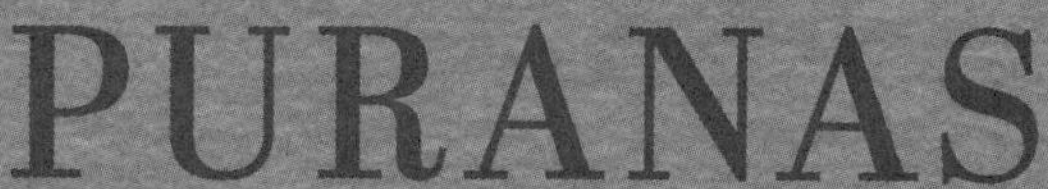

PURANAS

A Time Before Time

Beginning, Middle, and End– The Triad of Existence

Let's begin at the very beginning, delving into the depths of existence from unmanifest to manifest where the three energies of creation, sustenance, and dissolution (beginning, middle, and end) converge.

First we encounter Vishnu, the preserver, dharma upholder. His existence maintains the equilibrium of all life, harmonizing opposing energies. His resplendent, sky-blue skin and four arms cradle the world in a tranquil balance. This day, while walking on a narrow path engrossed in his duties and contemplating the profound wisdom of his teachings, he did not immediately notice the figure approaching from the opposite direction.

On the horizon, Brahma, the creator, the five-headed deity, drew near. Originally, Brahma had only one head, but his ardent affection for the goddess Saraswati inspired him to grow four more—one pointing in each cardinal direction—in order to keep constant vigil over her. Those close to Brahma were aware of his sense of superiority and arrogance for having created the universe.

Shiva, the god of destruction, was represented by a vast linga—a powerful representation of Shiva with a strong solid foundation holding a cylindrical phallic protrusion that pointed toward the sky. As Vishnu and Brahma approached each other, the path constricted, leading them to a pivotal point, the unpassable linga, representing Shiva. This linga was unusual in that it extended infinitely into the atmosphere above and its base descended down to the core of the earth. Disrupting their contemplations, Vishnu and Brahma looked up to acknowledge each other and the seemingly endless linga between them. After initial pleasantries wore thin, they each expressed their urgency to continue their journey.

With his characteristic arrogance, Brahma declared, "As I am the creator, you shall step aside and let me pass." Vishnu retorted, "I am the sustainer, maintaining balance and life in the world. It is you who must step out of my way and allow me to pass."

The two locked in a stalemate, agreed to a contest: Whoever could reach either the tip or the base of the Shiva linga first would be allowed to pass, while the other stepped aside. The contest was set, despite the obvious solution of one of them simply stepping aside. However, their stubbornness and hubris blurred the most apparent of solutions.

In a bid to win this test of dominance, Brahma mounted Hamsa, his swan, and soared into the sky to find the peak of the Shiva linga. Meanwhile, Vishnu began burrowing into the depths of the earth, tracing the length of the linga's base down.

As Vishnu descended to the depths, a profound frustration enveloped him. He knew with the unwavering certainty of his vast wisdom that the superior entity would have willingly and graciously conceded the path. Yet he continued digging and digging.

Meanwhile, Brahma ascended higher and higher into the sky, surpassing the clouds and leaving the atmosphere. With his five heads searching in every direction, he was intent on winning. Yet with each passing moment, doubt crept into his mind. An endless expanse stretched before him, and still the linga's top remained elusive. Fatigue and uncertainty threatened to overcome him, prompting thoughts of concocting a lie to deceive Vishnu.

In the midst of his inner plot, a gentle pink mallika flower descended from above, landing delicately in Brahma's open palm. Intrigued, he inquired of the flower its origin so high in the heavens. The flower, in its ethereal grace, responded, "A devoted soul placed me atop the Shiva linga, but a gust of wind swept me away."

Excitement coursed through Brahma's veins, as he assumed that the top was within reach. Eagerly he questioned the flower to ask if he had finally arrived, only to be met with its solemn declaration that he was nowhere near the pinnacle.

At this moment Brahma made a fateful decision. Overwhelmed by his desire to win, he decided to fabricate a tale. He instructed the flower to collaborate in his lie and tell Vishnu that he had indeed reached the top of the linga and plucked it from its sacred abode.

Back on the ground, Vishnu, weary and famished from his arduous excavation, conceded defeat, acknowledging that the linga was infinite, just as Shiva's cosmic role was.

On the other hand, Brahma returned with false bravado, brandishing the flower. He spun a tale about reaching the linga's top, plucking the flower from it, and meeting Shiva. Suspicious of this story, Vishnu probed the flower, which shyly confirmed Brahma's claim with an unconvincing "yes."

In that pivotal moment, a resounding boom echoed through the cosmos, causing Brahma and Vishnu to tremble. Shiva materialized in the wrathful form of Bhairava with a ferocity that shook the very foundations of the earth. With fiery intensity he exclaimed, "Liar!"

Brahma stood before him, his five heads wide-eyed, knowing he'd been caught in his lie. Shiva proclaimed, "Each one of us is pivotal in the balance of existence!"

In the wake of this confrontation, Vishnu, remaining in balance, continued along the path, as did Brahma, head slightly downcast from the reproach for his hubris. Shiva ascended back to his seat in the ether.

This profound encounter reestablished the indispensable nature of each entity's respective role, each with their own strength and importance in the cycle of life, no one winning or losing.

MYTH AND MEANING: THE ETERNAL CURRENT OF LIFE

As we journey back into the annals of time, into an era of divine beings and cosmic sagas, we do so not as strict believers in religious dogmas or deities, but as observers in the endless dance of life. It doesn't matter whether one believes in a god, or many gods, or spirits, or a divine intelligence, or in the exquisite power of nature. It's not even necessary to subscribe to a religion or belief structure.

These tales do not seek blind faith, but welcome those who embrace life's vibrant stream, a current flowing since the dawn of time.

Through the sacred triad of Brahma, Vishnu, and Shiva, we identify the faces of creation, sustenance, and transformation. Birth. Life. Death. Each deity has various avatars, meaning the deity's incarnation, manifestation, or embodiment into a new form. These forms offer us a lens through which to see our own inherent divine nature and the purpose with which we breathe life into this body in this lifetime.

The triad is a reflection of our journey and also reminds us of our impermanence. We're often fixated on the one-dimensional story of ourselves—our birth, our personality traits, and our ego story. Through the lens of these gods and goddesses and their avatars, we get a glimpse of our own multifaceted selves, transcending that which our eyes can see and our minds can grasp in our daily perception.

Brahma, the symbol of creation, creativity, peace, and honesty, save for this little hiccup of hubris in the story above. His divine consort is Saraswati, also known as Vac, who embodies the power of voice, knowledge, arts, music, and all creative endeavors. Together they are invoked at the advent of creative projects, musical pursuits, speeches, and whenever one embarks on a new journey. Notable avatars of Brahma include Valmiki and Vyasa, revered for penning the epic sagas, the Ramayana and Mahabharata, respectively.

Vishnu, the protector of justice, order, and mediation, personifies sustenance, along with Lakshmi who expresses abundance, prosperity, and grace. Together they intervene to restore balance when chaos and darkness threaten to consume the world. Lakshmi graces us with her divine vision, transforming the mundane into the extraordinary, and revealing beauty and preciousness in places where we perceive none.

Last in the triumvirate is Shiva, the embodiment of transformations, endings, and death. His energies encourage us to transcend the mundane, acknowledge the impermanence of our body, our personality, and our physical existence, and to find the infinite within. His consort, Shakti, a potent force of energy and power, inspires us to embrace the fluidity of life and live it to the fullest. This power couple embodies the forces of the finite and infinite. They simultaneously create life, dance feverishly through the cosmic theater, and celebrate the ultimate burning down back to dust. In this mythology the goddesses are not mere consorts, they're equal partners to the gods. They often hold the energy of action, bringing to life the intentions of their counterparts. Without Saraswati, there would be no knowledge for Brahma to begin creation. Without Lakshmi, Vishnu's sustenance would lack abundance and grace. Without Shakti, Shiva's infinite potential would remain dormant.

The feminine is an integral part of our existence. It guides us to balance our own masculine and feminine energies, integrating action with intention, and power with grace. It challenges us to rise above societal norms of gender roles, recognizing that we all embody these energies, regardless of our gender.

These representations of feminine and masculine, in the form of gods and goddesses, can assist us in navigating the intricate cycles of life—arising, experiencing, and surrendering, eventually to reemerge in a new form. Even as they change their forms and names, we can see each form expressing the qualities of their original essence. We see reflections of our own existence—our emergence, growth, moral quandaries, contemplation and attempts to understand the "why," and our surrender along the way until the eventual surrender to mortality. We recognize our weaknesses, attachments, and aversions, and the delicate balance between our egoic stories and our soul's longing.

Brahma's attempt to manipulate his way to being the most valued is reflective of what modern society celebrates. We celebrate the big win, the epic mountaintop, and sometimes, sadly, the chaos and division, often overlooking the simple, dedicated attention to showing up for life and sustaining honest connections. Social media and news bombard us with big, sensational trends, stories, dramas, and the things we "must" buy, missing the beauty of the mundane spaces in between all of the big stuff.

We are all within the structure of beginning, middle, and end at every moment of our lives, with one or two dominating at any given time. In this way, each of us carries within us Brahma, Saraswati, Vishnu, Lakshmi, Shiva, and Shakti. Our divine nature is always within us, waiting to be acknowledged and expressed. It is this inherent grace that allows us to empathize, love, create, and innovate. It allows us to navigate the complexities of life, using our discernment to choose the path of compassion and peace.

Recognizing our connection to these forces can guide us in embracing the different roles we play in our lives. It is in this dance of different personas that we express our essence in multiple ways, from the loving parent to the compassionate friend, and from the passionate artist to the inspiring leader.

The beauty of the puranas is not just in their colorful tales and allegories, but in the mirror it holds up to our humanity, revealing our divine potential. It encourages us to honor our journey, to celebrate our avatars, and to dance through the cycles of creation, sustenance, and transformation.

At the end of our lives, when we have danced through all our roles, when we have loved and lost, created and destroyed, learned and unlearned, we return to the infinite. We leave behind our transient form but carry forward the essence of our experiences.

In the words of the French Jesuit priest and scientist Pierre Teilhard de Chardin, "We are not human beings having a spiritual experience, we are spiritual beings having a human experience."

MYTH INTO PRACTICE: BALANCE IN PRACTICE

Mantra

Gurur Brahma.

Gurur Vishnu.

Gurur devo Maheshvaraha.

Gurur sakshat param brahma.

Tasmai shri-guruve namaha.

Creation is a teacher, stasis is a teacher, dissolution
is a teacher.

The teacher is Brahma, Vishnu, and the great god Shiva.

The teacher is absolute before your very eyes.

To that auspicious and revered teacher, reverence.

Meditation

Find a comfortable seat in any position that allows you to find a sense of length in your spine. Allow the breath to empty, then pay close attention as the breath streams into the body—the beginning of the breath. Move the focus next to the filling of the lungs as the breath nourishes and sustains the body. Finally notice the inevitable emptying of the breath from the lungs, out through the nose as the body is empty—the completion of the breath cycle. Keep your mind, body, and breath fixed on this cycle in its ceaseless repetition, experiencing the equal potency of each phase in this rhythm of life.

Movement

Sun salutations in the yoga asana practice illustrate a full cycle of movement, encompassing moments of opening and moments of release.

Begin in a standing position, like a mountain, then open your arms wide to greet the inhalation. Reach the arms up to the sky and bring the palms together, drawing this prayer gesture to your heart. Then begin to fold at the waist as the hands reach for the ground. Fold inward, then with an inhalation, extend your spine forward before stepping your feet back to find plank posture and lower to the ground. Inhale to lift your chest and heart forward and up, then rest the entire body with arms extended on the ground. Next place your hands back under the shoulders and press yourself to downward-facing dog, then step the feet between the hands and stand back up, arms to the sky, and return the hands to prayer position at the heart.

Explore three rounds of sun salutations with prostration, noticing the moments of openness, steadiness, and letting go.

Pay particular attention to the breath, and to the moment when one round ends and the next begins. You can also explore a modified sun salutation: Simply reach your arms out wide on the inhalation, then extend them overhead, connecting the palms, with a brief pause in the breath. Connect the palms overhead, then draw them back to your heart on the exhalation.

Exercise

1. In your journal, make a list with two columns. In one column list some of the ways you may avoid telling the full truth. In the other column list the feelings you experience when you stay in integrity and follow through with your commitment to yourself. Throughout your day, bring attention toward how you feel when you stay in integrity and grounded in the full spectrum of creation, sustenance, and destruction or completion.

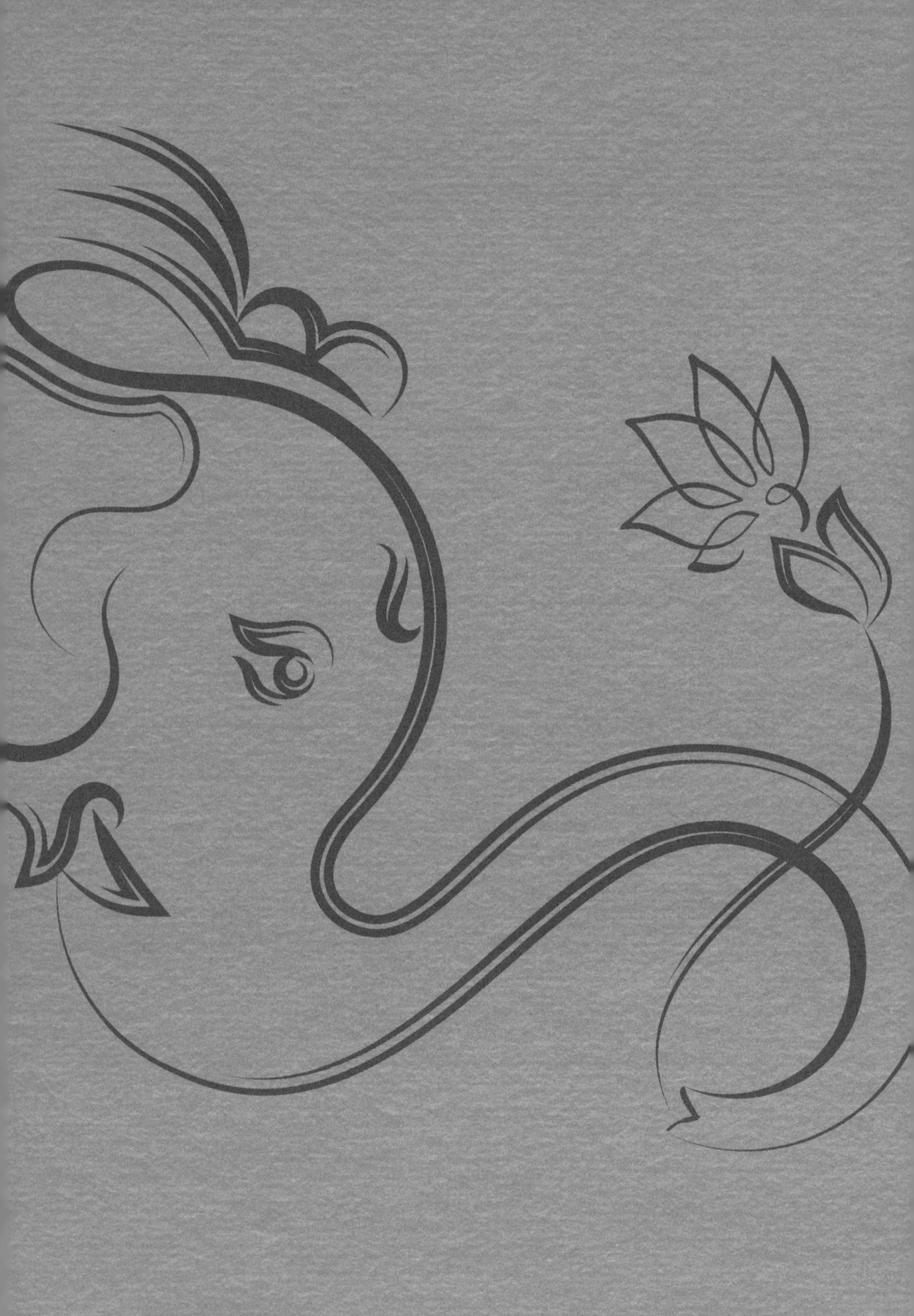

The Elephant and the Lotus

We find ourselves falling back in time to a small, remote village nestled high in the lofty Himalayas, an abundant and creative enclave brimming with artisans, craftspeople, and the most fertile land with unique and mouthwatering fruits and vegetables.

A place teeming with beauty, community, and history.

The village had just elected a new mayor, one with grand ideas to share the beauty and wonder of this community with the wider world. He had traveled extensively and had never seen any place quite as peaceful as his own village. Much like every good politician, he was filled with hope and innovative ideas that he believed would surely soothe the strife of the world through community and artistry. His enthusiasm to share the abundance of the village with those near and far was contagious.

The mayor thought long and hard about how to bring attention to this model village, which was built in harmony with nature and its inhabitants. After weeks of contemplation he was inspired to host a grand parade. He presented the idea to the townsfolk. It took some convincing, as some rightly preferred the village to remain a serene, undiscovered gem in the vast mountains. But because this new mayor's excitement was so contagious, the skeptical eventually relented and the planning began.

Months into the planning, the mayor began to feel like they needed a little something extra, an additional element of surprise. He began entertaining the idea of using the village's savings to purchase an elephant. This proposal took a bit more convincing, as the people wondered what they'd do with an elephant after the parade. You can return to silence after a noisy celebration, but how do you return an *elephant*? Nevertheless, the mayor's excitement was so compelling and his persuasive abilities so strong that the villagers finally conceded.

What shortly arrived in this quaint village was a vast creature that held the mystery of history in her tusks. With each resounding footstep, she lumbered into the hearts of the villagers as if they'd been waiting for her their entire lives. Every villager fell in love with this new friend, this symbol of celebration. They sought every opportunity to see her and bring her treats. In her presence, excitement for the parade began to build and a sense of pride began to grow. They named her Padma, as in the beautiful flower that signifies purity and spiritual growth.

The council spent countless hours deliberating how to adorn her, deciding when she would enter the procession, and settling on who would have the privilege of walking with her. But they spent *most* of their hours falling in love with her kind and endearing yet feisty spirit.

The newly elected mayor was thrilled. This had been his dream. It was the reason he had run for mayor. And his dream was coming true right before his eyes.

By the day of the parade, the villagers had decorated their main street, lining it on either side with stalls of fruits: the ripest watermelons, the juiciest mangoes, and the most luscious papayas. They set out tables adorned with vibrant vegetables, rich tapestries, precious jewelry, exquisite clothing, and delicious sweets.

As the dawn of the parade approached, every member of the village readied themselves, gripped with anticipation and exhilaration.

Then the rickshaws began to arrive. And arrive. And arrive. It turned out that the villages they had invited had in turn invited *other* villages, and so on. The turnout was astounding—beyond anything this small, remote village high in the Himalayas had ever seen. Everyone had heard about the elephant this town had purchased for their parade. She was extravagant, a mystery, and extravagant mysteries had a way of drawing people in.

The guests were warmly welcomed with songs from the local musicians, wafts of delicious delicacies, people in colorful fabrics streaming down the main street, and women in vibrant saris anointing them with a spot of rich red kumkum and sandalwood paste on their foreheads and garlands of fragrant flowers around their necks. As the villagers and their visitors gathered on the street in anticipation of the parade's start, whispers of excitement rippled far and wide.

At long last the procession commenced. Whispers swelled into excited murmurs as dancers floated down the street, followed by the most magnificently adorned rickshaws, rhythmic musicians, jubilant drummers, spiritual leaders, and more. As the parade grew, so did the sense of awe and wonder it evoked in its onlookers. But nothing compared to the collective gasp that occurred when the people saw the grandeur and grace of Padma as she turned the corner and showed herself for the first time. Each spectator marveled at her vast, magnificent elegance, feeling their hearts expand as they looked upon her.

Padma's body swayed softly side to side as she walked, her trunk affecting a hypnotic trance. She walked steadily and gently, like the old and wise creature she was.

But then something happened. As Padma arrived in the center of town, where the jewelry, clothing, and food stalls were lined up, something caught her attention: a ripe mango. Within seconds, the ceremonious Padma of the parade was but an elephant, desirous and unsatisfied. Before anyone knew it, she was charging toward the delicious treat. She saw no one and nothing but the object of her desire. Hundreds of people who had traveled hundreds of miles to see her were nearly trampled in Padma's fervent, single-minded pursuit.

Pandemonium ensued as her attendants scattered frantically in all directions, their cries piercing the air as the elephant's trunk finally made contact with the mango. But just as the fruit neared her mouth, a watermelon across the street caught her eye. What followed was a new desire, and as Padma hurtled toward it, more shrieks came from the onlookers, who were now unwilling participants in the chaos. People and animals fled in all directions, trampling one another in their desperate attempt to get out of Padma's way. Needless to say, the watermelon wasn't the end of it. Each time Padma turned her gaze, there was a new delight, and she ping-ponged across the town's main street, snatching up bunches of bananas, papayas, and more. Anything in her path was destroyed under her vastness as she surrendered to the desire for the ripe fruit all around her.

In the midst of this mayhem, the mayor had fallen to his knees, his head in his hands, as the villagers struggled to protect both their lives and their merchandise. The visitors jumped into their rickshaws and sped off to spread the word that this village was possessed by a crazy elephant, and cautioned others to stay away.

Eventually Padma had her fill. Her adornments smeared and her bangles torn, she wandered back to her pen to rest with an overfull belly. She rolled around in the discomfort of having gorged herself. As dusk fell and the quiet returned, the villagers slowly emerged from their homes to assess the damage. The mayor, on the other hand, retreated into his home, sinking into a deep depression.

After the proverbial licking of the wounds, the town council gathered to lament and to determine what had gone wrong. The meeting spiraled into a competition of who had suffered the most damage from the chaotic parade day. This, as one would imagine, went nowhere, as the mayor's apologies were drowned out by each council member's need to be the most affected, the most harmed, and the most put out by Padma's unrestrained desire.

Several hours into this cycle, after what seemed like an eternity, the door opened and in stepped the town elder, a reclusive figure who had lived sequestered in a cave on a nearby mountain for years. Without so much as a hello, the elder commanded, "You will send out invitations to all who attended the parade for a new gathering to be held in forty days." The room fell into a stunned silence. The proposition sounded utterly insane.

Soon a cacophony erupted, as all the council members began to speak at once. "That's ridiculous," they retorted. "No one will dare to come." "The previous event was a complete disaster. A destruction circus. This will be yet another one." "We are already ruined." The elder, in response, raised his right hand in the gesture of fearlessness—the *abhaya* mudra— silencing the room once again. Unwaveringly, he reiterated,

"You will send out invitations to all who attended the parade for a new gathering to be held in forty days."

In this humble village, the unspoken rule was clear: The elder's decree was final. The mayor snapped out of his wallowing, and with no small amount of unease, the council, along with the townspeople, dutifully set to work to honor his command and hold the event again.

The days ticked by and the invitations went out. But this time, instead of a stream of RSVPs, the neighboring villages remained silent. Crickets could be heard.

Meanwhile, deep in the mountain wilds, the elder settled into the rhythms of guiding the elephant Padma back to herself, channeling the wisdom of his teachers and all the teachers that came before, generations of those who selflessly shared the dance of teacher–student and student–teacher. All of the colorful delights of the world still remained, and the elder noticed and appreciated this. Yet, as the elder walked the paths of forest delights with Padma, he worked on pulling Padma's senses back in and grounding them in a deeper place.

Day in and day out, the elder gently led Padma through increasingly tempting distractions, constantly guiding her focus to a single point. The structure of their days evolved into practices to support her in picking up and holding something delicate in her trunk, something that would steady her. If someone were to observe this daily routine, they'd find it elegantly simple, tender, and consistent. Together, the elder and the elephant would rise early, forage for morning treats, and then begin the practices. Trust grew between them, and their rituals grounded them both in the *eka drishti* (single focus) and the inherent beauty within.

No one from the village knew what the elder or Padma were doing during this time—and not for lack of effort. Despite their attempts, the villagers caught no glimpse of the duo, and this fueled wild rumors. He had set her free. She had escaped back into the wild. He was seen riding off to the horizon with her. And so on.

On day thirty-nine, the mayor, who had now lost large chunks of his once lustrous hair, whose eyes were now sallow, and whose clothing was rumpled, was seen chewing his nails down to the cuticle, sweat dripping from his brow. As dusk fell, the villagers set up their stalls along the main street—this time with trepidation, each looking at the others as if to ask, "Are we *really* doing this again?" Fear prompted them to place their stalls farther from the street in the hopes that this time God would keep them safe. No one knew if anyone would show up after the utter disaster of the previous event. Up until day thirty-nine, the response to the invitations had been a resounding silence.

Not a single villager slept that night. Wide awake under the vast mountain sky, they imagined all the possible scenarios and felt fear stirring in their hearts with every beat.

The next morning the clouds parted, opening the blue ceiling of the earth. Roosters crowed, birds chirped, fragrant smells wafted through windows. The sun burst into the eyes of the sleep-deprived villagers. The day was beginning—whether they were ready for it or not.

As the villagers took their positions, and as they readied the procession, the fruit stalls, the flowers, the savory treats, the hand-woven blankets, the saris, and the tapestries, they looked around with uneasiness. Still there was no sign of the elder. Still there was no sign of Padma. Still there was nothing but the deafening silence among the villagers and at the core of their individual fears.

Finally the first rickshaw pulled up, and out stepped curious onlookers. The rumors of the catastrophe had spread, and they wanted to see this one for themselves—after all, everyone loves a good story. Moments later, a second rickshaw showed up, followed by a third, and then another, and another. To their astonishment, the villagers looked down the road and saw rows of rickshaws and travelers lined up to enter the village. Curiosity had won over common sense, and the village filled up with even *more* people than it had during the first parade.

As the crowds amassed along the street, the people cautiously stood back just a little bit farther than the last time. They wore running shoes. They wore looks of excitement and fear in equal measure.

Finally the parade began—*again*. New songs, new dances, new exotic animals fell into step along the way, and the onlookers clapped and danced. But they constantly kept one eye focused down the street, anticipating Padma's arrival—if Padma ever chose to show.

At long last she arrived, rounding the corner adorned in magnificence. Just as before, she emanated grace and wisdom. And yet the villagers knew they had fallen for this before, so it was with a tense awe that they let out gasps of wonder. Padma had taken only a few steps before the onlookers noticed something different from the last time—the elephant's trunk was wrapped around a lotus flower, held directly in her gaze. They watched her marvel at this lotus—held with a delicateness and reverence unusual for an elephant—as she walked. As Padma moved through the crowd and approached the fruit stalls, some onlookers became tense with apprehension. But others didn't. Something about Padma with the lotus looked so very different that they relaxed into an incredible sense of trust.

With a *different* form of single-mindedness this time, Padma strolled the entirety of the village's main street, lined with all the same ripe and delicious fruits and surrounded by the same array of temptations. Yet somehow she didn't seem to notice them, and remained undeviating from her calm center. She sauntered with elegance and composure.

What had changed? Just a lotus flower?

What only the elder knew was that he'd spent every day of the last forty days and every night of the last forty nights with the elephant, training her to notice the lotus, to take delight in it, to tend to it, to listen to it, to observe and honor its beauty and power; to see it as new in every moment. Like sadhana, or daily practice, Padma was gifted the quality of attention that allowed her to become free—free to not trample on people and things in her pursuit of momentary sensory delights. Free of the stomachache of overconsumption. Free of the incessant disappointment after obtaining each new fruit she thought she'd wanted more than the last.

Padma's steps were steady as she moved past the fruit stalls, her trunk curled gently around the lotus. The villagers stood with bated breath, waiting for the familiar crash of destruction, but it never came. Instead, her gaze stayed fixed, her movements calm, and a quiet rippled through the crowd that felt as extraordinary as the songs and drums that had opened the day.

By the time Padma reached the far end of the street, the village was unchanged, every offering intact. The elder walked forward to join her, and together they turned toward the mountain path. A hush lingered in their wake, the villagers watching as the great elephant disappeared into the hills, the lotus still held in her grasp. Long after she was gone, that stillness remained as if the flower's presence had taken root in every heart.

MYTH AND MEANING: POWER OF ATTENTION

Elephants carry the powers of history, time, lineage, and the earth's wisdom. As highly sensitive and intelligent creatures, elephants have inspired a sense of awe. We humans hold them as a symbol of a time span we can only attempt to imagine. Their vastness is humbling—so much so that it has evoked in some a desire to control these majestic creatures, to make them objects of entertainment, or more frequently to kill them as a misguided means of alleviating the sense of the insignificance their grandeur evokes. And so we have brought this fifty-five-million-year-old species to the brink of extinction.

The disconcerting fact that the elephant is teetering on oblivion due to the unchecked desires of a species (yes, us humans, who are, at most, three hundred thousand years old) is one reason this story resonates so deeply. Trampling over everything in our path, the human species has lost its lotus flower and appears to ping-pong from one shiny object to the next. We think we're reading a tale about an elephant, but in fact we are being exposed to ourselves in the mirror of the story.

The result of this heedless conduct is heartbreak, profound disillusionment. We're missing the nectar that's right in front of us by crushing everything in sight, wreaking havoc in our pursuit of things that are ultimately empty—*stuff*, excess stuff that often leaves us feeling even more desolate and dissatisfied than we were before we single-mindedly lunged for it.

In this story, the elephant represents our naturally graceful and inherently grounded nature; yet her unchecked and undirected desires in the market exhibit the way our senses pull us off our center and, more devastatingly, incite us to trample others in our quest for the next desire. When we begin to covet or long for something, we often become owned by it. And as we become possessed by that which we desire, we fail to take into account the ripple effect this has on our own well-being—much less the well-being of the greater whole.

When we see something we want, the brain, the body chemistry, and our *samskaras* (deep-seated emotional imprints) get to work, and before our resolve or good sense knows what's up, we're grabbing at the thing we crave. We abandon our center, trampling everything in our path in our rush to reach this elusive thing. In a frenzied rush to obtain it, we leave all sense of integrity behind, crushing biodiversity, the earth's resources, someone's feelings, other's freedoms, and whatever else is in the path of our momentary desire. You'll notice that in this story, Padma never takes a moment to revel in the taste of the mango before she lunges for the watermelon. Such is the nature of unchecked, uncontrolled, and undisciplined desire. It disregards all there is to be present for and ignores what's here to be grateful for. It doesn't just trample over *others* to get what it wants, it also tramples over what we already *have*. As we walk through the market of life, we're always lunging at things: partners, status, money, security, symbols of our success. We rarely stop to consider what we're hurting and what we're avoiding within us as we grasp for what we think we want.

The gift of the practice of sadhana lies in noticing, in acknowledging what is here, in the present, in the *now*. The story teaches us to seek and discover a profound inner connection to our source—our dharma, our life's purpose—and to stay true to it. We traverse the inner terrain to find a still point, a point of focus, a locus we return to again and again, keeping our eyes on it as the market of life attempts to pull us down shadowy paths, promises of more, and lanes of distractions. In doing so, we avoid looking at the ceaselessly changing nature of impermanence, our own mortality, and our discomfort with the apparent polarities and paradoxes of human existence. We numb the intensity of being embodied, and the suffering of *samskaras*, karmas, and imprints that drive us.

Temporary pleasure is a powerful, albeit ineffectual, medicine. A wonder drug. But if we persist as puppets to our ever-shifting desires, we will never experience peace.

The true gift of consistent practice lies in narrowing the incessant habit of being pulled in all directions by our senses. *Drishti* is the practice of narrowing our gaze to a focal point to turn the attention of the mind inward. In the story, Padma is named after the lotus, which symbolizes this *drishti*. Padma the elephant carries the lotus before her as a guiding beacon, an object of reverent attention. For us, this focal point can come in the form of a deity, a candle, a breath, a spot on the wall, a grain of sand, a creative project, or a loved one. *Drishti* doesn't even demand our eyes; we can also practice using a sound, a taste, a smell, or fusing all our senses into a multidimensional field of awareness. Ultimately, the external *drishti*—the directing of the senses at objects in the world in order to focus our attention—is a tool to bring the spotlight inward to the true central focus. This is the great paradox. *Drishti* looks outward at the phenomenal world to draw us back to our true nature, our center, to the one who is not chasing the drama wheel in that same phenomenal world.

It's often not until we zero in and concentrate on ourselves that we become aware of how scattered we are otherwise—our minds flitting from thought to thought, distraction to distraction. In asana practice, we often rest our gaze on a single point to provide literal balance. The balance that shows up in the body when we focus our gaze is analogous to the inner balance we long for in the entirety of our being when we practice focusing our attention. Through practice, we unify all of the seemingly disparate bits of the human experience into one grain of sand, and then back out again to the entirety of the universe.

In the practice of *drishti*, we embark on a journey defined by the fifth and sixth limbs of Patañjali's Yoga Sutras: *pratyahara*—drawing in the senses; and *dharana*—concentration, or bringing attention to a point of focus.

Whatever we focus on is where we expend our prana (life force). By softening our grasping energy and turning inward toward a deeper awareness, we cultivate more intimacy with the present moment and infuse more integrity into our life's course. It is a more wholesome way to use our life force than to live in a state of distraction and craving—precisely as depicted by each element of the story.

The mayor is our expression of ambition, the wish to externalize what we carry inside, to manifest our inner world externally, and to share it, inviting others in for the good and bad of it all. He represents our longing to connect and be seen. His role in the story shows us the disaster that this desire to exhibit ourselves can produce, as well as the grace that the desire for connection can invite. When tended to mindfully, this aspect of the self can push us past our comfort zone and into the scary but rewarding world of self-expression. However, when left unchecked it can create a pretty big mess.

Padma's lotus represented the *hridayam*, the spiritual heart. It is a reminder of the beauty and skillfulness inherent in single-minded focus, of a life lived in honor of what is *within* us rather than what is outside of us. It recalls our interconnectedness to all living things, emanating from deep in the earth, ascending up through the stem of our body and into the blossoming light of our hearts, and shining into the world with our uniqueness. The lotus serves as our tether; it is whatever helps us rein ourselves in, enabling us to walk through our human existence with grace and dignity. Its flower signifies purity, but a purity that roots into the mud and muck of existence for growth. Thus the lotus represents any of the tools available to us to bring ourselves back home to the landscape of our inner awareness. As we withdraw our senses from the shiny world and direct our gaze to the lotus of breath, meditation, or any other centering tool, we transition from the fifth to the sixth limb of yoga—*dharana*—and rest in contemplation.

Finally, the elder symbolizes our inner guru or a teacher who pulls us back onto the path and is willing to sit with us and spend those forty days (or forty years) by our side, constantly reminding us to turn our gaze toward the lotus. The teacher, whether within us or outside of us, guides us from darkness toward illumination (the word *guru* literally translates to "dispeller of darkness"), toward what truly matters. With help, we can access the wisdom gained through sadhana, this diligent practice of continually bringing our attention back to our intention.

This tale embodies the commitment to return to our core essence. To melt through the nearly constant longing-and-aversion cycle, and be present with the sacredness of the moment that is right in front of us. Ninety-nine percent of our suffering would fade if we stopped obsessing over things that are yet to happen or things that have already happened, and if we made a ritual out of attending to the lotus of this moment. Sadhana is our human attempt to ritualize our lives. In the practice of yoga, it's the attempt to move through all of the cycles of resistance, boredom, ego thrashing, and the all-pervasive belief that the world needs us desperately and can't do without our worry or attention for five minutes or it will fall apart. Because these, too, are the mangoes and watermelons we're lunging for.

Sadhana is the daily effort to turn our attention toward our lotus, whatever that means for each of us. For some, that may be the heart; for others, the divine, grace, or God. Regardless of the form our lotus or our *drishti* practice takes, it allows us to return to the beauty of simplicity. Whatever the lotus is for each one of us, it is in a sense our inner light—a place in the midst of the placelessness of external ups and downs, wins and losses, which, when attended to, guides us to our essence, to our true self.

As I walk through the marketplace of life, I can smell, touch, taste, hear, and see all the wonders and horrors, yet stay centered. I don't have to retract from the richness of life nor be constantly ruled by my preferences and distractions. I can notice how delightful it is not to be pulled in all directions. I can pick up a mango, taste it, and revel in what it means to be in a body with taste buds that spring to life *without* longing for more.

The fruit in this story is not a symbol of something we are supposed to sidestep. It is the material phenomena we get to delight in for the short time that we inhabit these bodies. And this practice of staying delighted in the moment is a continuous work in progress. I can't merely set the flower in place and be done with it. I have to continually bring my gaze back from the chaotic physical world, reassemble my mind to the heart of things, and balance the internal world with the external.

However, when I do this—when I slow down and notice what's right in front of me, and that it's enough—I realize that I am also enough.

MYTH INTO PRACTICE: PICKING UP THE LOTUS

Mantra

Om mani padme hum.

Praise to the jewel of the lotus.

Meditation

Visualize a lotus flower at your heart. Draw your *drishti* (gaze) to this imagined flower and feel your breath come and go, as if the breath provides nutrients to keep this flower alive and the flower the nutrients to keep you alive. Settle into the earth and feel its solid nature below and within you. When the mind begins to wander, patiently bring it back to the flower at your heart. Notice every sensation of the flower—its texture, fragrance, colors, stem—and keep coming back to it as if it's real and right there.

Movement

Close your eyes and try to balance on one foot. Then open your eyes and look all around. Lastly, find a clear spot to focus on. Push into the earth through the standing foot, and notice the power of *drishti* to support your balance.

Exercises

1. Write down three things you could do instead of lunging for distraction in order to keep your attention on your lotus flower.

2. Write down what brings you back to your center? Pay attention throughout the day when you lose sight of it.

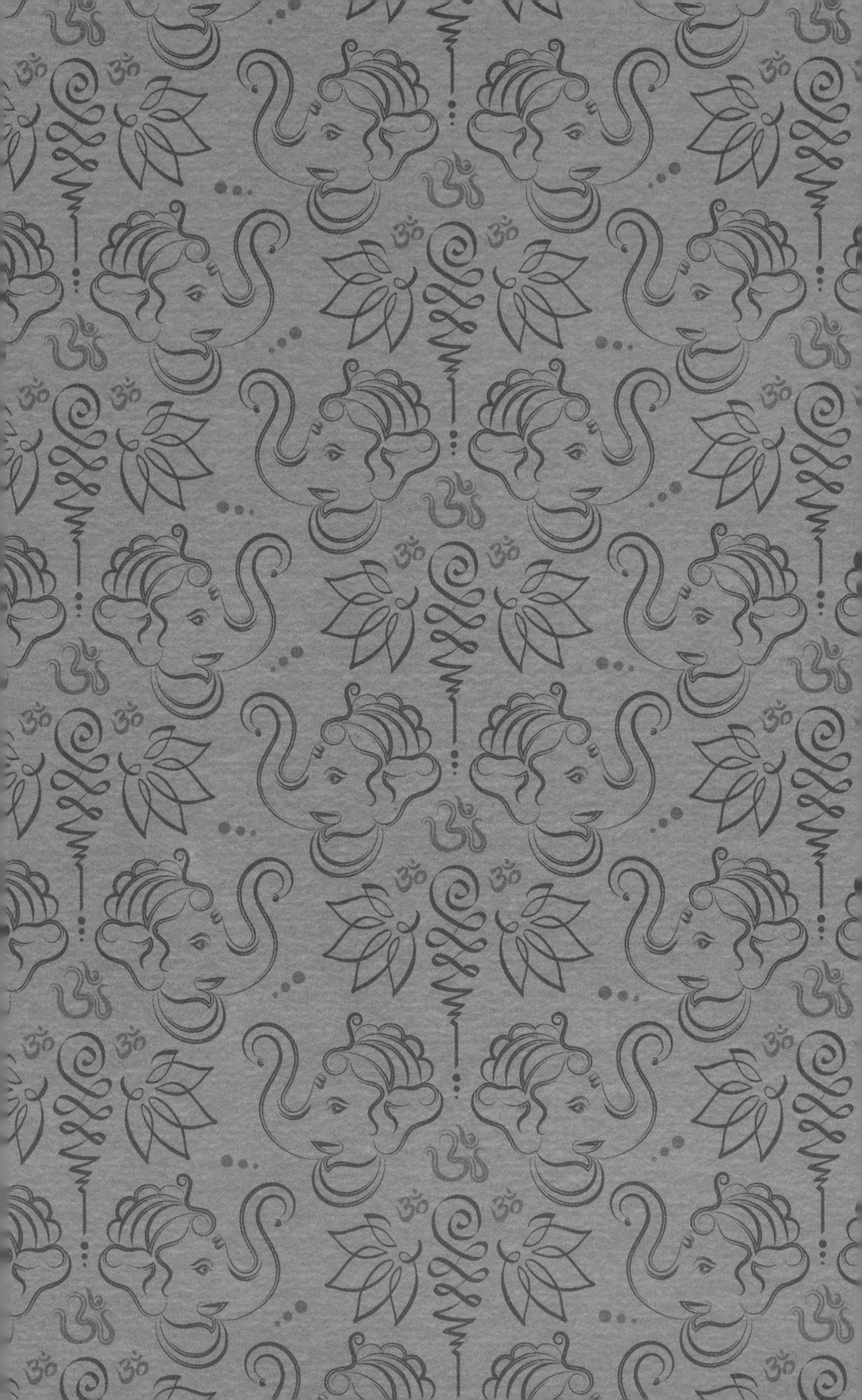

Ganesha—New Beginnings

We find ourselves in a time before time itself came into existence, high up in the magnificent Himalayan landscape of Mount Kailash, where the power of nature thrusts toward the heavens, reminding us of our humble existence amid its grandeur. The sacred peak of Mount Kailash has long been regarded as the abode of gods and goddesses, a place where divine energies converge and spiritual seekers embark on transformative journeys.

Our journey to the majestic, sky-high summit unfolds with the enchanting Parvati, the elegant mountain goddess and loving consort of the almighty Shiva. Parvati represents the creative and nurturing aspects of the divine feminine. Her grace and radiance illuminate the mountainside, attracting all those who behold her presence.

The union of Shiva and Parvati is one of divine balance, of finite and infinite, feminine and masculine, the sun and moon.

Shiva was once an unlikely candidate for marriage. However, even this cosmic dancer and destroyer of illusion found himself captivated by Parvati's magnetic allure and unyielding determination to transcend the celestial realm and experience the human facets of partnership and family. Unable to resist her relentless perseverance, the all-powerful Shiva ultimately conceded, and their heavenly union was formed.

Their union transcends the boundaries of time and space, reflecting the eternal dance of the cosmos. It symbolizes the inseparable nature of opposites, as Shiva represents the formless and transcendent aspect of existence, and Parvati embodies the manifest and intrinsic forces that give rise to creation.

However, despite the fulfillment of her matrimonial wishes, Parvati's yearning remained unquenched. She longed to bring children into existence and experience the boundless love of motherhood. Shiva, however, dismissed her desires as trivial pursuits reserved for the mortal realm, where *avidya* (ignorance) and suffering abound. He argued, "Why would you bring anything into the world that is going to die? Why would you add to the suffering?"

Nonetheless, Parvati's longing remained pure and strong. While Shiva traversed the cosmos, creating worlds and spreading the teachings of yoga, he was oblivious to the stirring emotions within his own home. During one of his many journeys, Parvati, in her daily ritual of waterfall bathing, invoked her longing. Bringing forth her unwavering desire and intertwining her love for Shiva with his love for her, she manifested a miracle: From the divine fusion was born a beautiful son, a testament to the power of their eternal bond. She called her child Vinayaka.

Shiva continued on his celestial journeys, lost in time and space, leaving behind his beloved—now a single mother who was raising their remarkable son alone. She nurtured him with utmost care and love, infusing him with strength and wisdom. With time, this beautiful child blossomed into a young lad—an embodiment of his mother's fortitude and father's spirit.

Parvati continued to honor her sacred ritual of daily respite. In the same secluded spot where she had manifested her son, she would cleanse her body and soul while losing herself to the rhythm of water, washing and anointing herself with exotic oils that perfumed the mountain air. She entrusted her son with guarding her privacy. It was his duty to stand guard at the entrance every single day during her sacred bath and divine energetic communion with Shiva, and Vinayaka fulfilled this duty with unfaltering devotion.

One day Shiva returned home to his wife, his beloved. He had been married to Parvati for thousands of years—many, many lifetimes—so he was well aware of her daily ritual. As he approached her bathing sanctuary, he was met with an unexpected sight: a strapping young man standing guard. He commanded this young man to step aside. The young man without hesitation refused, responding, "No, you may not pass." Since Vinayaka had never met his father, he didn't know whom he was stopping; all he knew was his duty and responsibility to his mother and that he would never fail her.

Shiva found this amusing. "Who is this fool who stands between me and my beloved? Does he not know who I am?" After some back and forth, he soon realized the seriousness of this young man's intentions. He was not going to step aside, and Shiva's amusement turned to jealousy and rage. Incensed, Shiva unleashed his immortal fury, blazing with rage and directing his mighty *ganas* to attack. The *ganas* were no ordinary army—they were a group of men so skilled, so formidable, that they'd never tasted defeat before. They were the virtual embodiment of man's sensual experiences, known to overpower adversaries with their fierce resolve. However, the tables were turned in this encounter.

The five senses—smell, taste, sight, hearing, and touch—each attacked Vinayaka, who valiantly confronted this onslaught with his innate wisdom and inner strength. In an unprecedented act, he vanquished the invincible *ganas*, bringing them down to their knees.

With his army strewn on the ground before him, Shiva was taken aback. No one had ever defeated the powerful *ganas* before. Who was this extraordinary man who dared to defy him? He failed to understand that this young man was his own flesh and blood.

Shiva's bewilderment soon turned to wrath, leading to a fierce confrontation between him and Vinayaka, and a great battle ensued. Father and son both desired to protect Parvati, yet were unable to see through their pride and understand that they were on the same team. The combat was fierce and Shiva was startled by this mere mortal's power. Shiva's frustration exploded, and in an act of finality he pulled out his *trishul*—a three-pronged spear—and decapitated his own son.

Alarmed by the commotion at the threshold of her bathing chamber, Parvati emerged hurriedly, her divine self drenched in essential oils and elixirs, and adorned with flowers, precious minerals, and turmeric paste.

Before Parvati stood her dearest Shiva, his towering presence casting a shadow on the headless, lifeless body of her sweet, cherished son.

A shriek of pure despair exploded from her core, so devastating and heart-wrenching that Shiva felt a tremor threatening to dissolve his celestial existence into the ether. The harrowing wail pierced through the realms, drawing in the concerned villagers, who swiftly gathered around.

With a surge of determination to undo the damage, Shiva sprang into action, leaving for the lower realms in search of a suitable replacement head for their son. There he encountered Gajasura, the ancient demon elephant who carried the burden of a timeless curse to roam the earthly realms. Sensing an opportunity for liberation and redemption, Gajasura willingly offered his head—a selfless act of sacrifice through which he could attain moksha and live eternally, adorning the divine form of Shiva's son.

Hastening back to his son and beloved wife, Shiva's heart raced with anticipation and hope. Taken aback by the sight of an elephant's head, Parvati let out a fleeting screech. However, as the elephant's head nestled upon her son's delicate shoulders, a divine metamorphosis unfolded before her eyes. The revived son of Shiva and Parvati arose from the ground and people from far and wide gathered around as the proud parents anointed him with the name Ganesha, the remover of obstacles and the beacon of new beginnings. On his feet, Ganesha stabilized himself with his new head, and soon an expression brimming with uncontainable joy erupted on his face, as he playfully raised his trunk and began dancing.

Parvati's fears disappeared, giving way to profound relief as she watched her husband and son dancing together with boundless love and harmony. The scene was a wonderful embodiment of creation and destruction, a celebration of impermanence and eternity, and a testament to the eternal wisdom and the unbreakable bond that unified them as a divine family.

To this day Ganesha is one of the most beloved and famed deities in the Hindu pantheon.

MYTH AND MEANING: BEGIN AGAIN

As the story of Ganesha unfolds, we find ourselves bearing witness to the transformation of this powerful deity as he adorns various guises, reflecting our own journey through the earthly and spiritual landscapes. From his birth as Vinayaka to the emergence of Ganesha, the elephant-headed god, he was known by many names. Ganesha was also called Ganapati—the lord of senses, as he was able to tame the senses. He was also known as the lord of new beginnings and nature's history keeper, and each role has profound significance. Often called by the affectionate version of his name, Ganesh, he is a relatable deity with whom many develop a personal relationship.

In his birth as Vinayaka, we perceive the harmonious balance between the masculine and feminine energies within us. Parvati, representing the feminine, embodies the power of nurturing, creation, and intuition. It is she who kindles life, feeding it with love and care, nurturing it from seed to bloom. Shiva represents the masculine, and embodies strength, detachment, and spiritual wisdom. His energy is a tempestuous force. Their divine union and Parvati's subsequent ability to manifest the birth of Vinayaka serve as celestial mirrors reflecting our own journey toward our inner strength.

Parvati's longing to manifest life from her divine union with Shiva serves as a compelling reminder of the profound power that lies in our own internal equilibrium. This equilibrium is a delicate dance between surrender and action, the finite and the infinite, and the transient and the eternal. The harmony between these contrasting forces within us is the creative force itself. It is the pulsating life force that shapes our essence, a source from which all creation springs, just as a lotus blooms from murky waters. Whatever we create, forge, or give birth to is a reflection of this inner divine balance. The act of creation isn't just a physical act, but a transcendental journey of self-realization that guides us from the finite constraints of our existence to the infinite realm of spiritual consciousness.

Before becoming Ganesha, Vinayaka the protector stands guard at the threshold of cleansing, where his mother purifies herself, and where abundance and sweetness manifest through Lakshmi. His role as the steadfast protector highlights the need to safeguard our personal spaces, the sanctums of our mental and emotional well-being. In our everyday lives, this translates into protecting our time and preserving boundaries. It teaches us the value of carving out moments for self-care and rejuvenation, for the nourishment of our soul.

As the lord of senses, Ganesha battles the senses that incessantly assault us. He emerges victorious time and again, demonstrating resilience in the face of adversity. The modern world, with its ceaseless stimuli, often causes an onslaught on our senses, stirring feelings of being overwhelmed and, at times, anxious. In these moments of sensory overload, we can learn to navigate the turbulent waters of our sense cravings without being swallowed by the waves.

As humans, we often react unconsciously in violent ways when we perceive that our senses are assaulted. The feelings of disgust, annoyance, or anger that erupt within us are born out of a sense of being overwhelmed, or underlying fear. Our primal instincts are powered by this potent emotion. Often we operate from very old programs wired by evolution and passed down from our ancestors. When we pause to investigate deeper than just the immediate reaction, we may observe that our anger or fear stems from that old wiring. Peeling back the layers of fear, unmasking its capacity to spark violence, and understanding the frustration it fuels when we feel powerless, this deep understanding helps us better comprehend our reactions.

By understanding our relationship to our sense preferences, we don't need to suppress them as much as work with them. By awakening to our senses, we learn to leverage them to unearth the sweet nectar of life. By being mindful of our sensory experiences, we learn to adapt to them instead of letting them dictate our reactions.

Ganesha's wisdom extends beyond the realms of our senses. He teaches us to cultivate resilience, focus, and inner fortitude to rise above our challenges and distractions with grace and clarity of purpose. With conscious engagement and understanding, we can use our sensory experiences as tools to experience the richness of existence.

Though the story of Ganesha momentarily veers toward sorrow, redemption blossoms on the horizon. In his atonement,

Shiva replaces Ganesha's head with that of an elephant, the keeper of wisdom and history, the sustainer of nature's chronicles. This transformation echoes in our lives, reminding us that obstacles and challenges are not roadblocks but catalysts for growth and transformation. As the lord of new beginnings, Ganesha reminds us that each breath we take, every dawn that breaks, and every communication we embark on is a chance for a fresh start, a new beginning. Even moments of unkindness can sow the seeds for transformation, providing us an opportunity to engage with more compassion and kindness.

True growth and self-realization often require us to let go of old identities, beliefs, and attachments, and to embrace new possibilities with an open heart and mind. Ganesha's story encourages us to see transformation as a natural part of our spiritual journey, and accept the unknown with trust in the process of personal evolution.

Empowered by the history-keeper wisdom of the elephant head and pure-earth body, Ganesha is said to have used his tusk to write the Mahabharata, an epic text that serves as the root of many of our profound teachings, including the Bhagavad Gita. By understanding and mastering our senses, we too have the ability to uncover a wellspring of eternal wisdom. By transcending the impulses of our senses and harnessing our energies, we can access the depths of insight and knowledge that reside within us.

Within Ganesha's realm, we are encouraged to embody the qualities of childlike wonder and curiosity. In our fast-paced and often serious adult lives, he is a reminder to reconnect with the joy of simplicity, spontaneity, and exploration. By cultivating childlike wonder, we can approach life with a renewed sense of awe, openness, and a willingness to learn. We immerse ourselves in the symphony of experiences, finding beauty and magic even in the ordinary moments of life. This curiosity fuels our thirst for knowledge, our desire to explore uncharted territories, and our unwavering belief in the boundless opportunities that await us. With Ganesha, we embark on a transformative quest, where every obstacle becomes an invitation for growth, every change an opportunity for self-discovery.

Ganesha serves as a reminder that we can begin again and again and again, as long as we have breath, and that within each of us lies the potential for immense growth, strength, and enlightenment.

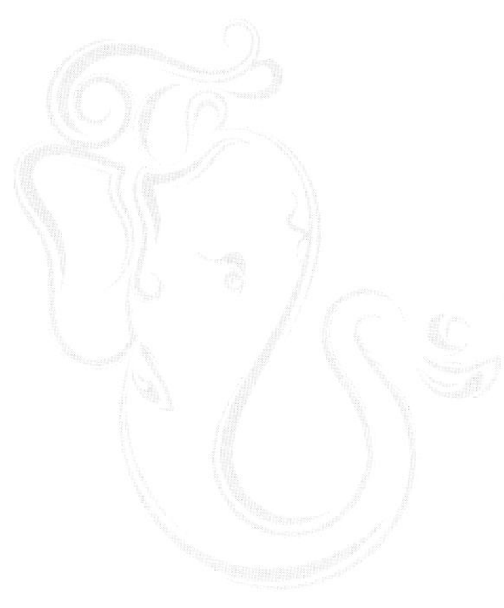

MYTH INTO PRACTICE: BEGIN AGAIN

Mantra

Om gam ganapataye namo namaha.
Invocation to Lord Ganesh, the remover of obstacles, who guards the doorway to the enlightened realms. His blessings for good beginnings.

Meditation

Find a relatively quiet place for this meditation. Close your eyes. After a few deep breaths, begin to notice the quality of light, even with your eyes closed. Explore bringing your attention to the light and then withdrawing your attention. Next, notice the sounds around you. Allow any judgments of sounds to pass through your mind without clinging to ideas about what is a pleasant sound and what is not. Just allow all to be sounds, and let them wash over you. Now notice any smells that waft by, again letting go of judgment and allowing them just to be. You can stick out your tongue and notice if there are any subtle tastes. Pause again, pulling all of these sensations back into your being. Now notice the sensation of the clothing on your skin, and of the air on your skin. Attend to the temperature, any movement of air, the stirring of your clothing if there is wind. Rest in this attention, again without judgment. Take a few more deep breaths, pulling your attention back to your whole sensing being.

Movement

With your feet on the earth, barefoot if possible, move slowly with steady groundedness. Keep returning your attention to the feet and your relationship to the present moment.

Exercises

1. From a standing position, with knees lightly bent, draw up onto the balls of your feet, then drop your heels to rapidly descend to the floor. Repeat this ten to twenty times. Pause, stand still, and allow the reverberation from the ground to pass up through your body.

2. Is there a person, circumstance, yourself, or situation you could see through new eyes? Journal on the ways you would like to use the practice of beginning anew to change your perspective on this situation.

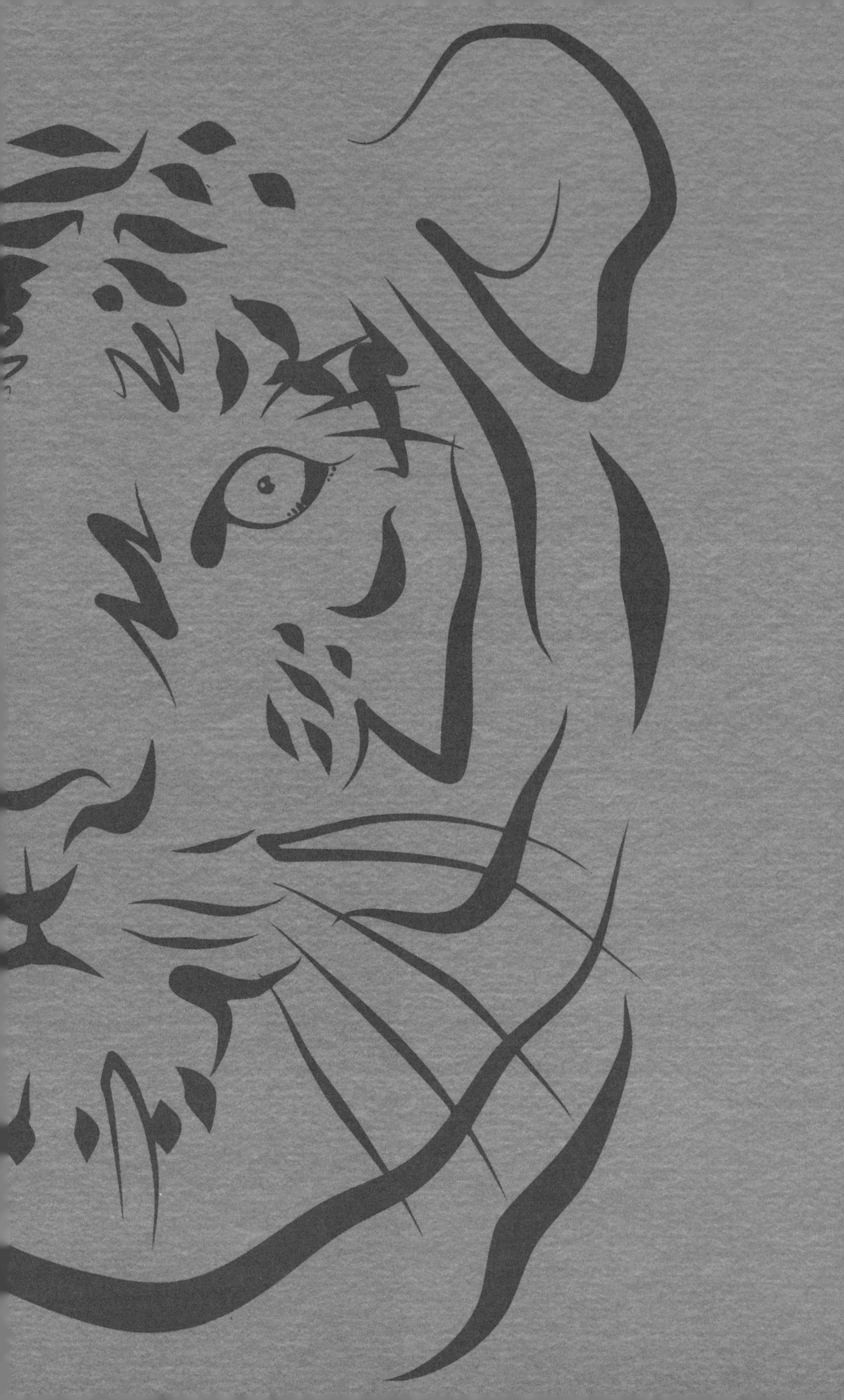

Durga—Fierce Compassion

As we journey through the tumultuous expanse of time, we descend into a period of great disharmony and darkness across the earth, when the theater of existence was taken over by a demon, or asura, named Mahishasura. Known as the buffalo king, he terrorized all who encountered him, with his horns protruding from his skull, his fangs, and his fierce fiery eyes. He had become so power hungry and malevolent that his poison leaked across the lands.

His unchecked greed, fear, tyranny, and deception were given center stage, feeding power to this negative energy that rippled into everything. The world slowly adopted fear and mistrust as a way of being during this dark time. Mahishasura's rule brought out the worst in everyone. The shadow realms took over, forcing kindness, love, compassion, and community out of the world. Just like that, there was simply no room for these virtues.

As the veil of darkness descended, it went unnoticed by most adults, who were immersed in their own scrambling to get more, have more, be more. The draining of love and compassion from the world was so slow and so subtle that they went about their tasks oblivious to the transformations both without and within. It was the children, with their open hearts and wide-eyed awakeness, who first noticed the changes. They noticed the weakening of the smiles on the adults' faces. They observed how their parents' brows grew heavier, how aunts and uncles began to speak of others in hushed and harsh tones. They perceived how suddenly every adult action stemmed from a closed-hearted sense of fear, or distrust, or even malice. But most of all the children noticed how the sweets and fruits of the earth began to dry up. How even the dirt no longer nourished them.

While the adults, with their myopic attention on adult things and their gradual mirroring of Mahishasura, remained insensible to the change, the gods and the devas—like the children—soon registered the transformation. The gods watched as their devotees turned to the pursuit of power and money, rejecting their previously heart-centered actions. They watched as neighbors eyed each other with suspicion. They held their divine breaths waiting for burnt offerings, for the ripples of reverence that used to emanate from temples and homemade altars, enriching the community with kinship, friendship, tenderness, and human love.

But then the gods found themselves holding their breaths for a very long time.

Flashing back a few thousand years, this corruption began with misguided devotion. Mahishasura had been a humble student of Brahma long ago, long before he morphed into a demon and took the name Mahishasura. He had initially dedicated his life to serving the power of creativity and creation. To demonstrate the strength and degree of his reverence for Brahma, he undertook an intense ritual. He underwent a strict fast, standing on one foot under a tree for many years, praying. This painstaking ritual eventually extended for centuries, until one day, Brahma, overcome with delight at this show of faithfulness, decided to pay his devotee a visit.

Bursting with pride and thrilled with the attention he received, the student proceeded to ask Brahma for a boon. His ask? That neither man nor god would be able to slay him. Curious ask, Brahma thought, but even the gods are swayed by flattery. Brahma considered all those centuries the asura had stood on one foot for his sake, and each of the prayers that the asura had prayed rang in his ears. And he agreed to Mashishasura's request. The moment Brahma acquiesced was the moment he fell prey to his own pride. "There you go," said Brahma to Mahishasura, "I give you your unslayability—by man and by god."

The moment Brahma nodded his head and granted his boon, Mahishasura transformed from a faithful disciple to an omnipotent tyrant, growing more and more powerful, more and more untouchable, as the days went by. And so began the interminable, insatiable hunger for power. The asura's features morphed from those of a strong, lithe human devotee into a raging, strong buffalo man, and he took the name Mahishasura, the buffalo demon. He discarded his former friends, surrounding himself with those who starved for the scraps of his power feast.

When the gods and devas discovered that none of them could touch Mahishasura because of the foolhardy, ill-considered boon, they furiously confronted Brahma, who had since lost interest in the small dramas of the earth and its creatures. Brahma was forced to acknowledge his blunder. But now the gods had to plan quickly. Back on earth, those few who had held onto kindness and right action (dharma) as guiding lights were forced into hiding. In Mahishasura's kingdom, it was no longer possible for them to live uprightly in public. Their love, their benevolent acts of kindness, their very humanity had become a threat to those who succumbed ever deeper to their demon nature. Those who did not go into hiding were persecuted by Mahishasura's followers for their generosity of spirit. Mahishasura's followers were lost in their demonic transformations, nearly unrecognizable from their former selves.

The gods searched frantically for a divine loophole in Brahma's boon. They sat around a raging fire, day and night, seeking to burn away misperceptions, return to clarity, and uncover a solution to the conundrum. For one hundred and eight days, the gods sat at the fire, eyes closed, mantras flowing. On the one hundred and eighth day, they opened their eyes to a divine spectacle: the most radiant being emerging resplendent and effulgent, out of the center of the flames. It was Durga, arising with her ten arms unfurling with strength, her hair aglow, body firm and upright, lit from every direction. Her presence swept across the gods' and devas' faces with such power and force they all sat awestruck, unable to move. One of the gods, Shiva, instantly recognized his other half—the Shakti to his Shiva. Her face was exquisite, open, and magnificently awash with compassion, discernment, and pure, unclouded focus.

That neither man nor god would be able to slay him, Mahishasura had asked. But of course, the asura's appeal to Brahma had mentioned nothing about a woman, a divine goddess in pure feminine form.

The gods gasped in awe at Durga's fierce clarity. The dormant energy that had been recently awakened was not messing around; she was laser-focused and ready. This was no simple errand. This was the calling of Durga. With an immaculate combination of fierceness and compassion, Durga hopped on her tiger, grabbed the many weapons her many arms could carry, and with barely a nod to the awestruck gods she took off, leaving nothing but a trail of smoke behind them—the lingering sense of a divine burning. With a sigh of relief and an excited anticipation, the gods gathered themselves up to watch the unfolding of this goddess in the face of a demon none of them could battle.

Durga's journey to the gates of Mahishasura's kingdom was swift and direct. Standing at the seemingly impenetrable doors, she steadied herself and her tiger, grinding deeply into the dry earth. Inside, the kingdom stirred with a mix of apprehension and excitement.

From his high tower, the demon was transfixed by what he saw. Blinded by his colossal ego, Mahishasura believed that this extraordinary woman had traveled all this way because of her desire to offer herself to him. His minions were thus dispatched to escort her in. But when they opened the gates and stood face-to-face with Durga, they were nearly brought to their knees, overwhelmed by her grace, by the power of her beauty. They couldn't quite recognize that what they saw in this visitor was an unfaltering but loving resolve to act in the face of injustice.

Instead, they saw her as an object of desire. Knees still shaking, they carefully informed her that Mahishasura had agreed to take her as his—though even as they did, some of the minions suspected that Durga was too powerful to have arrived with such an intent. Durga's face remained steady, open, and calm as she spun her web, informing them that in her kingdom, it was customary to battle with potential lovers to determine their worthiness.

Mahishasura, upon hearing this, scoffed at the idea. Why should he, the mighty one, waste his energy fighting a woman he would soon own and rule? Refusing to stoop, the asura commanded his entire warrior army to battle the visitor. What a pity, he mused, to decimate such beauty—but then again, they weren't exactly dealing with a being of compassion, and the pang subsided nearly the moment it arose.

The assembled army approached the gate, preparing to take this beautiful flower of a woman and crush her as ordered. But as the gates swung open, what happened next surprised everyone except the gods, who had witnessed Durga leap from the flames on the hundred and eighth day and advance into this battle with a fierce resolve.

The army stormed toward Durga with their weapons drawn, armor secure, and fury in their eyes. Durga, compassion still emanating from her eyes, raised her ten arms with their ten assorted weapons, and within seconds, in a blur of divine activity, she vanquished the entire warrior army.

Amid the applause of the gods, shock descended upon Mahishasura and his shadow kingdom. Shaking off his rage, the tyrant assembled his most notorious warrior, Raktabija, and sent him out to the kingdom's threshold, to the gates where Durga stood calmly amid the carnage. Raktabija arrived at the gate filled with arrogant confidence, ready to demolish this petite woman with ease. Once again, the kingdom gates swung open as they looked on, this time with a little more trepidation. Before them stood Durga, upright, magnificent, serene, and alert.

Captivated by her demeanor, Raktabija found himself unnerved and swallowing hard. What is that astonishing look on her face? he asked himself. It's something that feels a little like tenderness, almost like love. But the feeling wasn't enough; he was too deep in the shadowy trance of Mahishasura. Mahishasura loomed in the distance behind him, and he felt his ruler glaring at his back. He shook off that uncanny feeling and marched forward.

Raktabija was startled by Durga's swiftness, her deftness, her unimaginable ability to be in multiple places at once.

However, Raktabija, whose name means "he for whom each drop of blood (*rakta*) is a seed (*bija*)," was confident.

As Durga approached him, her many arms flying, slashing at his flesh with her blades, each drop of blood that fell from the warrior penetrated the dry, barren earth. And each drop of blood that came in contact with the earth became a seed that gave life to a new Raktabija. This way the warrior multiplied exponentially, until the battlefield was soon swarming with a vast and growing army of replicas of Raktabija, all clashing with the goddess.

From the safety of his chamber, Mahishasura watched in the distance as thousands of Raktabijas spread across the field. He howled and puffed his chest in delight, failing to notice that Durga had closed her two eyes and was battling this army of Raktabijas blind. From between her closed eyes a small opening began to appear, unbeknownst to the Raktabija army. This aperture in the middle of Durga's forehead slowly widened until a formidable and terrifying body exploded from Durga's third-eye center: the goddess Kali.

When Kali raged onto the scene, it was with pure, wild fury—her tongue extended out, her eyes rolling back in her head. Kali arrived as we know her: hair turbulent, a skirt of arms wrapped around her waist, a mala of skulls draped around her neck—the arms and skulls remnants of all those she had liberated from earthly attachment, from the hypnotic grip of egoic delusion. Kali's third eye was wide open, filling everyone who witnessed her, including the mighty Mahishasura and the inhabitants, with a profound sense of awe and dread, goose bumps across every inch of their skin. With utmost clarity in every cell of her being, the goddess began to perform two terrific tasks at once: She annihilated each of Raktabija's replicas with her wild hands; and with her tongue she caught every drop of blood that fell from their bodies before it could touch the parched earth, preventing the creation of more Raktabijas.

Had you been near the battlefield that day, you would have watched, open-mouthed, as the army of Raktabijas disappeared before your eyes, until only a single Raktabija remained: the original one. But you would have had to watch without blinking, for a moment after there was only one Raktabija left, that Raktabija was gone too. Unceremoniously Kali consumed him. After all, there is no time for ceremony in the life lesson of detachment.

With the opposition obliterated, Kali turned to her divine ally and immediately retreated back into Durga's third eye. Durga, perched on her tiger, was now the sole figure facing the gates of the evil kingdom.

Silent and awestruck, every inhabitant of the kingdom wondered the same thing: What would their ruler do now? As they slowly found their feet and remembered their voices, they assembled at Mahishasura's doorway. Gathering strength in their throats and in their fists, they began to persuade their leader to face this unknown woman at the gate, this enigmatic woman who'd just annihilated the very warriors whose duty it was to protect and conserve the greed and deception that motivated every facet of their lives, that justified their power. The pressure came not only from Mahishasura's minions, but also from his court. "What a coward you now look like, hiding in your chamber, Mahishasura," they derided.

The tyrant offered a series of limp excuses for his reluctance to face this tiger-riding woman. He too had seen something in Durga's eyes—a force that he knew he'd have to face, a force that he feared might utterly change him. Indeed, a force that might bring him to his knees in its mild ferocity. But he had built his reputation on his unslayable nature, on his immunity. Mahishasura had no choice but to uphold this egoic burden he had built for himself.

Mahishasura had grown weak through centuries of exploiting his minions, forcing them to do his work for him. He gathered his weapons and his remaining courage, pushing through the assembly with his public performance of self-righteousness, which by now had built into a scream. He boasted that this would be the briefest and most astonishing battle they'd ever seen. This stranger at the gate was but a puny girl who'd gotten lucky in those first two battles. No, it wasn't even luck—she must have cheated. She knew nothing about the man she had to face next—his boon, his vigor, his immortality.

Tucked inside the most extravagant and costly modern armor money could buy, Mahishasura roared up to the gates, which were promptly opened for him. As he stepped with one foot over the threshold of his kingdom, he looked—for the first time—directly into the face of his opponent, and for an instant his entire body seemed to go limp. He gasped audibly, as though he was outside of himself. Before him stood the most magnificent creature he'd ever seen. From afar he hadn't noticed the exquisite grace that emanated from Durga's being. He hadn't wholly experienced the peacefulness of her composure, the quiet certainty with which she held herself. Most importantly, he'd missed that fierce compassion in her gaze. Like his second wave of soldiers, Mahishasura now recognized in Durga's eyes something he had known in his former life: a courageous promise to uphold what is just and good, a calm commitment to standing firm in the face of inequity. But above all, a tenderhearted gaze that upheld that commitment—even as she looked upon the asura whom she would have to slay.

As the crowd roared, Durga stood in absolute grounded strength, unflinching at the overprotected figure in front of her. She could see the little scared boy inside the big, stiff armor. Her remarkable combination of benevolence and ferocity radiated across the land. Mahishasura, pressured by the cries of his subjects, charged bullishly at Durga. But with a simple sidestep, she let the asura rush past her and tumble to the ground like an awkward buffalo. And so the battle began.

It would be convenient to tell you that, as she'd done with the previous two armies, Durga quickly decimated Mahishasura and the day was won. But that's not the way this particular battle went. Durga pulled out the first of her ten weapons—the chakra, a spinning disk of potent condensed energy—and asura and goddess battled for a hundred years, blow for blow, righteousness against dishonor, until both combatants retreated to their corners to rest and recover.

As they rested and their eyes met, Durga fingered her next weapon. Then the battle commenced again. Another hundred years passed—blow for blow, purity against impurity and corruption. Each gained the advantage only to lose it again. Gods and devas wrung their hands. The inhabitants of Mahishasura's kingdom booed and oohed and ahhed. The intensity of the battle ebbed and flowed as the decades passed, yet inexplicably the ferocity of both opponents intensified. After a hundred years both collapsed into their corners to rest and regain strength.

Imagine this cycle of contests eight more times over. Asura and goddess clashed, again and again, more furiously with each of Durga's remaining weapons.

After the wielding of Durga's many weapons, Mahishasura and Durga fell into a state of complete exhaustion. Everyone now held their breaths, arms limp at their sides after centuries of hand-wringing. Mahishasura's minions stood on their toes, craning their necks to see over each other's heads. They pushed each other out of the way to get front-row views. What would unfold next? Mahishasura's shoulders grew broad and boastful. From his corner he smiled slyly at the goddess—the look of a man who thinks he's winning. At that signal, Durga began to rise slowly. She carefully mounted her tiger, her face as calm and open as ever. Was it possible, the onlookers asked themselves, that they even saw a hint of love in that face?

As tiger and woman strode toward Mahishasura, Durga lifted one leg, exposing the sole of her bare foot—a radical gesture of vulnerability. The demon king looked up, transfixed by both her loving gaze and her naked foot, both radiant in the light of the setting sun. Mahishasura gulped at this woman's self-exposure, certain that he had won, that this magnificent creature was now his to have and to own.

The tiger took step after step after step, and still the woman astride his back did not put her foot down. Each time a paw thundered against the ground, it brought with it a growing sense of excitement in Mahishasura about the imminent possession. As Durga approached, the earth trembled and exuded the scent of pure nectar. Arriving finally before the demon king, the goddess—still on her tiger, bare foot still exposed—looked down upon him with loving compassion. She gazed into and beyond his eyes, into and beyond his dark, heinous deeds. She saw the devastation and infinite suffering he had inflicted on so many, on the earth. Her eyes went soft as they connected with and validated the pain of those whom the demon had caused to suffer. And just as quickly some of the hardness, the resolve, returned to them. What returned was the firmness of necessary action.

As the object of that loving gaze, Mahishasura now remembered who he had been before he descended into the shadow world. He remembered himself as a pure being, devoted to Brahma, committed to creation and to generation, to kindness and to the relief of suffering. What happened? How did I get here? Who have I become? These internal questions occurred rapidly to him, but they were met with the same conclusion each time: I want relief from the demon who has taken me over.

In that instant, in the internal certainty of Mahishasura's desire, Durga's bare foot landed on his throat. The goddess reached into her belt, withdrew the *trishul,* her final weapon that she'd placed there centuries ago, and thrust it downward, into Mahishasura. As death overtook him, Mahishasura felt only a deep exhalation: the freedom of release from what had forced him into his shadow nature with its accompanying greedy pursuits. Like taking off a binding and poisonous suit, the asura returned to his simple, humble self. All that remained was a plea for forgiveness and a prayer for love to replace the darkness.

Durga took neither pleasure nor pain in this act of compassion. Nor did she rejoice in her victory. It was simply her dharma to release Mahishasura—as it was her dharma to release all beings—from the grip of delusion that creates a sense of separate subjects and objects, of us against them. Mahishasura returned to his natural form, merging back into union with the infinite. As for the inhabitants of his kingdom, they began to awaken from their shadowy stupor, remembering compassion and kindness, reviving their commitment to equality and justice.

In the midst of this remembering, her job now done, Durga mounted her tiger and set off into the fiery sunset.

MYTH AND MEANING: FIERCE COMPASSION

When Durga makes her first appearance, she is seen rising from the radiant fire, ablaze, illuminated, and burning with lucidity. Her ability to sit in the fire and gain strength from it rather than be consumed by it is a striking testament to the profound clarity that comes from our own burning, our own personal trials, from the willingness to endure the fire of discomfort, to melt and change and be transformed.

The steadfastness in Durga's emergence from the fire, mounted on her tiger, is an expression of precision and clarity of mission. There is zero waste of energy or time on superfluous fluff or frivolous niceties. With the knowledge of what awaits her and the weight of this mission, she is ripe with purity of purpose.

Durga comes forth when we're done with the people-pleasing, when we stop dancing around matters and give up trying to manipulate a situation passively. She signifies the moment when we're ready to confront situations head on, with directness and determination.

Durga is known for her fierce compassion. Say that out loud: *fierce compassion*. How does it sound? Let's break it down.

When we think of the word *fierce*, we immediately think of ferocious, relentless, perhaps even rage. But it's what compels us to move away from danger or confront it. It's a mother's voice that grows sharp as they grab their child urgently to move them out of harm's way. The fierceness is as protective as a mother lion safeguarding her cubs. We witness it when we move out of a toxic relationship, stepping up for ourselves with a sharpness that cuts through old patterns. This is the power of the Durga energy—the power to use ferocity to move us away from danger and unhealthy patterns, drawing us into a deep well of strength.

Through Durga's relationship with her tiger, her mounting and riding it, we see a metaphor for harnessing our fierceness, our anger, and using it as power and strength. We often fear our own anger as we experience being out of control or lashing out impulsively. But when we learn to harness our anger and guide it toward necessary action, the anger becomes a catalyst for transformation. Mounted on her tiger, Durga is a manifestation of *focused* anger—an intensity that does not lash out in revenge or retribution against a particular wrongdoer or offender, but that holds justice, protection, and ultimate goodness as its guiding intention. In other words, fierce compassion is a power used *for* something, rather than *against* it.

This is the very force that can be drawn upon to make significant change in the world, as we see through protests and political, social, and environmental activism. This is the fire, the oomph, the driving force that gets us into action, mobilizing us from concept into motion. Often we find ourselves being against something, and this opposition could be channeled into creating something positive. However, many of us seem to get stuck in the anger *against*, failing to transition it into change.

Compassion (literally, suffering with) centers on connecting with the pain of others by witnessing it quietly and tenderly. It emanates from empathy and a longing to protect and support, and to confront injustice. In the story, Durga's gaze of compassion touches everyone who lays eyes on her, reminding them of the pure beings they once were before they got lost under their delusion and greed. Durga's ability to stand her ground (her fierceness) allowed her to sustain her knowledge of the greater good (compassion), even in the face of impossible odds.

She embodies the compassion of a mother—a mother who can witness their child making so many harmful choices but continues to hold them with compassion and love. It's the ability to see beyond the immediate action and into the suffering that causes this action. As Durga looks upon Mahishasura and all those around him who have caused pure suffering to so many, her heart remains open and she can see beyond their actions to the soul of their being. This is the compassion we *so* need in our current times, when division sells ad dollars, when outrage at one another is profitable, and when we deepen into an us-versus-them paradigm.

One of the embodiments of Durga is Gandhi—fierce yet peaceful, holding strong and true to right action yet focusing all of the fierceness born of injustices. Like Durga in the battle, he used every tool he could access, and had to keep falling back to regroup and begin again, eventually winning through vulnerability and fierce compassion.

Interestingly, the story begins with devotion, with Mahishasura as a diligent and dedicated student who gets a moment with Brahma. There's an initial innocence in Mahishasura, a sincere desire to learn, to undergo studentship and self-discovery through devotion.

But what Mahishasura misses when a delighted Brahma comes to pay a visit to his ardent devotee is that the objective of action is never the *reward* of that action. The reward is the action itself, as well as where our hearts are fixed as we perform it. This is a teaching given to Arjuna in the Bhagavad Gita, when Krishna explains to the warrior, "You have the right to work, but never to the fruits of work. You should never engage in action for the sake of reward." Krishna reminds Arjuna that everything in the world, except for his own actions, are entirely out of his control. If there is a fruit or a boon, it is the action for action's sake, and nothing more.

Ramana Maharshi offers this: "Do actions without caring for the results. Do not think that you are the doer. Dedicate the work to God. That *is* the skill and also the way to gain it."

Mahishasura overlooks the fact that he's already in possession of his boon—his practice, the only thing he can assert control over. The only agency he has is showing up, over and over again, day after day. It's all those years of fasting, of praying, of standing on one foot beneath the tree. It should not have mattered if Mahishasura's god *ever* arrived to show him his face because a divine vision is not the point. But the moment Mahishasura has access to Brahma, the logic of practice equaling reward is stirred within him. So he asks for a boon in return for his efforts.

Perhaps you've experienced this in your own practice and life; I know *I* have. I've forgotten that my faithful showing up—to the meditation cushion, to the next difficult but meaningful conversation—is all there is. There is no finish line to arrive at or ultimate goal to be reached. And if, in the midst of my practice, I trick myself into believing there is, I'm going to be sorely disappointed—because tomorrow will be a different practice altogether. We do not keep the fruits we think we've earned. This is why so many people abandon the path of practice, continually searching for an unattainable destination.

Mahishasura falls for this trap—except the buffalo demon gets his finale for a few centuries before learning the truth: Searching for fruits is an act of greed that perpetuates a false sense of ownership, a sense of deserving. And while the asura's greed manifests as an insatiable appetite for power, it is a rapacious and naive clinging to his own story, to the structures that might sustain it. *See this boon? It's divine proof of who I am, of what I deserve.*

This clinging to identity and entitlement is deeply rooted in *ahamkara*. In Hindu philosophy, *ahamkara* is the aspect of our psyche that identifies with the individual self, creating a sense of separation from the rest of the world. It is the ego that says, "I am this" and "I deserve that." It is the force that constructs and maintains our self-identity, distinguishing *me* from *them*. And while this sense of self is necessary for navigating the world, it becomes problematic when it dominates our consciousness, leading to egocentrism and a distorted perception of reality.

Ahamkara and greed go hand in hand. The more we feed the ego, the more it wants. This constant craving for more—be it power, wealth, or recognition—drives us further into a state of disconnection from others and from the true essence of life. The ego's insatiable desires create that perpetual sense of lack, fueling a cycle of wanting and acquiring that never truly satisfies. This illusion of separation and the relentless need to fill an internal void is what leads to suffering, both for ourselves and for those around us.

We see this in Mahishasura's story. His initial devotion and purity become corrupted with his desire for immortality and power, feeding his *ahamkara*. As he amasses more power, his ego grows stronger, creating a deeper rift between himself and the world. His greed and sense of entitlement isolate him, causing him deep suffering. His *ahamkara* makes him believe that his worth is tied to his power and invincibility. This separation from his true self and others generates fear, insecurity, and this constant need to defend his position.

But *ahamkara* doesn't just cause internal suffering; it also spreads suffering outwardly. Mahishasura's inflated ego and insatiable greed lead him to impose his will on others, creating an environment of fear and oppression. His sense of entitlement and need to protect his power at any and all costs causes widespread suffering, as his subjects are forced to live under his tyrannical rule. The ego, when left unchecked, becomes a destructive force that seeks to preserve itself by any means necessary, often at the expense of others.

Look at modern wealth and how it gets displayed, often gobbling up coastlines and resources in its insatiable greed. We can easily lose perspective in the maze of *ahamkara* and desire, and forget the point of life, love, community, relationships, and compassion. When we strive and finally get what we think we wanted, that can be when the spiral begins—we will defend what we've gained with whatever it takes to preserve it. Every gain—whether it's status, position, power, money, public praise, or recognition—becomes yet another thing to protect. And the number of things we might eventually be trying to hold on to in order to bolster our sense of self is inexhaustible.

Mahishasura gets his windfall boon but then lives beneath the thumb of its power, which is the great irony of this story, given that he appears to be the one wielding power. On the surface, the buffalo demon represents all that we see in modern-day autocrats, lobbyists, and corporatemongers, who tilt the system to stay in power, enriching themselves and their friends while leaving the rest to scramble for the leftovers. But more subtly, he represents *all* our shadow selves, with our quieter ambitions, selfishness, pride, and arrogance. And this ripples out to all spaces around us. This is where we need fierce compassion to confront and dismantle the toxic influence of *ahamkara*.

Durga enters the scene as the unequivocal answer to the gods' contemplation, after a hundred and eight days of conjuring a solution to the pervasive problem that is *ahamkara*, greed, fear, and decay of humanity. She emerges from fire—a force of transformation, where regardless of the fuel, the end result is ash. Fire represents *tapas*, the heat of discernment, the separation of nutrients from the waste, of illumination and the clarity that comes when we see beyond the veil of our illusions. If wielded with restraint, flames purify us, bringing us closer to our dharma, our lucid resolve. We sit in the fire each time we sit in meditation, each time we bravely and honestly look at our internal landscape and discern what's not serving us, each time we take on the challenge of burning through our thought patterns and unproductive habits.

After all, for fierce compassion to truly make a difference in the world, it must begin with ourselves. It's easy to read this story of Durga's battle as a battle between the self and the world's injustices and inequalities that we're called to challenge compassionately and courageously. However, we cannot find the power of that expression in the world if we don't first ride toward the demons of our own untethered minds, compassionately reining them in with all the weapons of practice we have available to us.

In my journey to understand or interpret these stories, I've noticed how easily I fall into binary thinking: Durga and Kali are good; Mahishasura and Raktabija are bad. However, what's worth remembering about this story (and indeed, about *all* of these stories), is that Durga's battle with Mahishasura is a metaphor for each individual's battle with our own internal nature, with our own shadow selves dominated by ego, greed, and selfishness.

The look on Durga's face—from the moment she emerges from the fire to the moment she places her bare foot on Mahishasura's neck and drives her *trishul* into him—is invariably loving, benevolent, equanimous, and composed. There's a motherly openness and receptivity to whatever she encounters along her path—as Krishna says in the Bhagavad Gita, "alike in pleasure and pain"—whether it's her beloved Shiva as she emerges from the fire, or the demonic power she's been called upon to wrestle with.

Remembering Durga's imperturbable face reminds me to pay attention to the tension patterns in my own face, the expressions I display when confronted with something or someone that sets my dislike trigger off. Unclenching my jaw is a step toward softening and remaining open. It's about becoming receptive to what arrives into my life, and *how* it arrives: my children, my colleagues, my friends, my antagonists, the gifts in my life, and the deaths and challenges. Leading with a soft face when I encounter conflict or difficult moments is one small way to stay open to all aspects of experience. Durga's unwavering compassion is a practice of a lifetime; but starting here, with the mask I wear to protect myself from the world, is a meaningful beginning.

Along with a soft face, Durga also possesses a third eye on her forehead, just like Shiva. Although hers is usually imperceptible, it opens in times of need, and we get to witness this moment when it expands, allowing Kali to spring forth. Kali doesn't waste a moment, as she is the power of time and time is coming for all of us. Time is coming for all our possessions, our beliefs, our bodies. Time will bring us all back into the earth, and we shall all be reconnected by Kali, by time.

During our brief journey in this body that has us believing we're separate from everything, we will all eventually end because of Kali. Her skirt of arms represents her ability to release our grasping and clinging one way or another—the nice way or the cut-off-the-appendage-that-is-holding-on-tightly way. She wears a necklace of skulls, representing the delusions of the mind that she will snatch away too. The riddle of Kali is that she will come for these things gently, but if you're clinging to your attachments, she will most likely rip them from you.

This shows up in humans' insatiable appetite to take, dominate, own, and devour the earth's resources, and Kali symbolizes the myriad of signs and warnings along the way that urge us to readjust. And when we don't pay attention, she comes with raging fires, floods, bomb cyclones, and other catastrophes. Yes, these are the manifestations of natural laws and science, but the energy of Kali is within them.

When we cling to a relationship, job, or old story, when we can't seem to let go, when our *ahamkara* becomes unchecked, this is often when the energy of Kali comes in a more abrupt and violent way, cutting it off, incinerating it, and somehow clearing it away.

Kali is detachment, and she reminds us that the material world and all the stories and identities we believe constitute the I/me/mine are not certain. Kali is a persistent reminder to unclench our hands and accept what falls into them, because what falls there is sure to go; what arrives is sure to depart.

Kali's arrival comes at the moment we confront the deepest roots of our attachment to our stories, illusions, smoke-and-mirror games, and our own Raktabija—our ability to evade the simple truth of our mortal, impermanent being. We change our diet, we cultivate discipline, we kill one of our demons, only to have another sprout from it. The true power of Kali manifests in turning and walking toward the full obliteration of our grasping, controlling, managing, and manipulating self. She is always ready—her tongue out, eyes rolled back, hair ablaze, ready to receive me when I resist humility, or she comes as an infinite purple space when I surrender, when I'm humbled and I quit resisting.

After wielding her many weapons, Durga exhausts all of them, leaving her empty-handed. In the final battle, Durga mounts her tiger, face soft and open, and purposefully exposes the base of her bare foot. It's a gesture of utter vulnerability, of absolute surrender. At times, we too must put our tools down and simply walk nakedly and fearlessly toward ourselves—toward our deepest demons and our darkest secrets. We must walk, completely toolless, weaponless, defenseless, knowing that we will discover both darkness and light there, and that one is not better than the other; knowing that we must love what we discover in that naked-looking being, all while holding a face of compassion and fierceness expressed in that naked vulnerability.

In the end, this vulnerability is all we have. We must set down our defenses, strategies, and management tools to enter the final threshold, to walk directly toward what we fear the most, to arrive at the sacred dwelling of the heart.

This walking-toward-ourselves with love, acceptance, vulnerability, and compassion is an act of pure *sraddha* (faith); it is the faith in both ourselves as our own resources and our own teachers, as well as in our practice to light up some intuitive work within us. It's the opposite of ego—where we look at ourselves in our pure vulnerability, without a mask of someone we think we should be, without the armor of our false stories.

Durga can be vulnerable precisely because she's so secure in her purpose, because, after eons of standing in the fire's heart, she knows her internal landscape so well. All she needs is within her.

MYTH INTO PRACTICE: APPROACHING THE DEMON

Mantra

Om dum gurgayei namaha.

Invocation to goddess Durga and the fierce compassion energy to protect me from the shadow forces.

Or:

Om mata om Kali Durga devi namo namaha.

I bow to the mother and her expressions as Kali and Durga.

Meditation

Find a comfortable place to sit and ground your body and take eight deep breaths. Bring to mind a current challenge you're facing right now. Bring it fully into view with all its accompanying feelings. Notice if your breath shifts or your heart rate increases. Bring your face into a calm, soft, and open expression, embodying Durga: your body upright with strength, riding your tiger, barefoot, exposed, and facing adversity. Allow your face to rest in the expression of fierce compassion. Notice what it feels like to approach that challenge on the tiger, Durga-like, with simultaneous vulnerability and clarity of purpose. How does becoming Durga change your relationship with the challenge?

Movement

Infuse your movement with heat, clarity, and fierce compassion. Use the power of discernment to listen internally to where you feel shame, fear, or resistance.

Remember Durga's face and hold that look in *your* eyes and face when you can. Can you find softness in the more challenging movements? Can you hold with compassion what arises as you move your body into certain positions? Can you keep your palm open, face soft and able to be vulnerable *because* you're so secure in your purpose?

Exercises

1. What elements of your life demand more compassion or more ferocity from you? Take one item from that list at the end of the day, and spend the following day taking steps toward transforming your relationship to that element.

2. Ask yourself if now is the moment you need to hold the sword of discernment, or is it the time to be vulnerable. Maybe it's a difficult conversation that needs to happen, or a boundary you want and need to draw. Can you take the first step toward creating that moment?

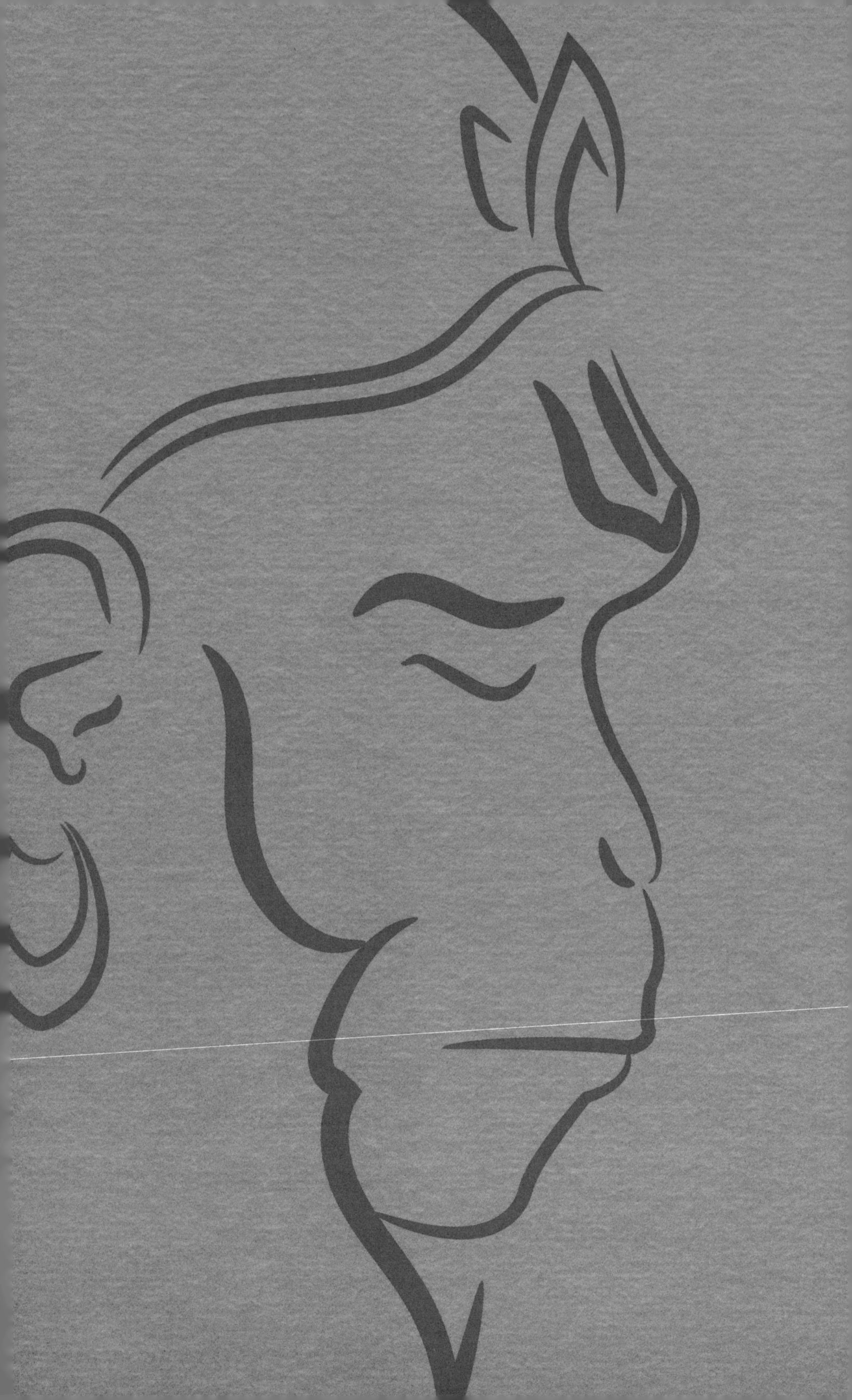

Hanuman—Superpower

We begin in the presence of the exquisitely beautiful, vivacious, and proud, Punjikasthala. She resided in the palace of Indra, the god of heaven, lightning, thunder, and the sun. Despite the opulence of her existence, she grew bored and restless, often yearning for something more stimulating than the routine comfort and luxury she experienced.

One day, in the pursuit of some amusement, Punjikasthala descended to earth. While in the forest, she encountered a monkey in deep meditation, sitting in lotus pose as though he were a man. She chuckled under her breath. *Was this a joke?* She couldn't believe that a monkey could sit so solemnly, wild-haired, like a human sage. The sight tickled Punjikasthala so much that she began to giggle louder and louder until she burst into peals of thunderous laughter.

The meditating monkey, however, remained undisturbed. Unaccustomed to being ignored—for she was the center of attention wherever she went—Punjikasthala soon grew annoyed by the monkey's serenity and repose and started throwing things at him to grab his attention. She threw stones. She threw flowers. She threw fruits. The monkey ignored this pummeling for as long as he could, until a particularly big rock hit him just below his heart, making Punjikasthala the object of his wrath.

With his patience gone, the monkey opened his eyes, turning them furiously toward her. This was when Punjikasthala realized that she had been tormenting no ordinary monkey, but rather a sage—a divine saint who'd only taken the shape of a monkey so he could better concentrate on his absolution. He sharply reprimanded her: "Your stones and fruits have disturbed my meditation. Your youth and beauty have made you snobbish, causing you to treat others like careless beasts. You do not yet know how transient both youth and beauty are. So that you may one day understand your transgressions, and because you are now acting like one, you will take the form of a monkey on this earth in your next life."

The thing about a curse from a sage is that it can't be retracted; once the words are uttered they're irreversible. So while Punjikasthala begged for forgiveness, raining her remorse upon him, nothing could be done about her next life as a monkey-faced woman. But the sage's heart melted a little as he witnessed her sorrow, and his anger subsided. He consoled her, saying, "Do not despair; in spite of your monkey face you will be deeply loved and respected. You will bear a great son—a divine monkey child, an incarnation of Shiva himself—who will become known as the greatest of devotees. And after you bring him into the world, you will be relieved of your monkey form and returned to your celestial self."

When the time came, she was reborn as Anjanay, a monkey huntress. Over time she met and married the monkey king Kesari, the ruler of Sumeru, and led a mostly happy life. But a vague memory of her prior celestial existence lingered with her, reminding her that her present earthly life was the consequence of a curse. This faint remembrance of her former celestial grandeur left her feeling that her current form, with her long tail and sharp teeth, was somewhat beneath her. So she lived a life of intense spiritual practice, fervently worshiping Shiva in the hopes of bearing the prophesied son who would liberate her from her curse.

In response to her devotion, Shiva finally appeared, granting her desire for a son through Vayu, god of the wind. Vayu carried the seed of Shiva and implanted it into Anjanay, leading her to blossom into the fullness of maternal anticipation. Her delight and excitement for a son eclipsed any desire to escape her circumstances. Soon enough she birthed a little monkey boy. They called him Anjanaya (son of Anjanay). With the powerful love and protection of his mother, the wind god, Vayu, and the monkey king Kesari, Anjanaya flourished and grew strong.

In fact, he grew stronger than the other boys—and very quickly. He outpaced his friends in every race and outmatched them in every sport, every game, every contest. His friends watched in awe as each new day Anjanaya grew noticeably stronger, more able-bodied, more powerful. His friends begged him to do tricks: to become lighter than air; to fly over walls of dense forest foliage and retrieve their balls and lost toys. They asked him to shrink down to the size of a particle and sneak around to eavesdrop on exciting conversations. They urged him to manifest the objects of their desires (typically sweets of some kind) out of thin air. They did not focus on Anjanaya's vast differences from them. Rather, they fixated on what they could get from him.

The adults, on the other hand, noticed Anjanaya's behavior and grew suspicious. While he did not intend it, his play wreaked havoc in every corner of the village and beyond. He knocked over trees by simply leaning on them. A careless kick as he was walking propelled massive boulders into a river, changing its entire course. He'd often shriek with laughter, and the air that burst forth from his lungs in these moments changed the ocean tides. Ruled by his frenetic monkey mind, and with no real awareness of the degree of his strength, Anjanaya unwittingly left a path of destruction in his wake. The surrounding villagers began to complain. To defend his son,

Kesari argued in a kinglike fashion, "He may look different from the other boys, but that's just his princely nature."

One morning Anjanaya was up early as usual, with as voracious an appetite as ever. Stomach rumbling, he looked up searching for the very best mango he could feast on. Every fruit he laid his eyes on looked far too small to satisfy the appetite of his growing monkey body, until he caught sight of what appeared to be the most gigantic, ripest, most scrumptious-looking mango he'd ever seen: the sun. Driven by the sprightliness of his ravenous, childish desperation, the monkey crouched and leaped with a force that sent him soaring beyond the trees, past the birds, through the clouds, and finally out of the earth's atmosphere.

Anjanaya found himself flying past asteroids with zero interest in anything other than that ripe, delicious mango above him. He was salivating, as if he could taste the juicy sweetness already. In his singular focus on his desire, he failed to notice that he was heading directly toward the sun.

Suryadeva, the sun god, was blazing peacefully in the sky when he looked up and saw the figure of a monkey hurtling toward him like an arrow. Suryadeva watched, taken aback, as Anjanaya grew bigger and bigger as he came closer—much, much bigger than a man. This was a first. Uncertain of what to do with a rapidly approaching enormous monkey, mouth wide open as if he were going to consume the entire sun, the sun god let out a cry for help.

Upon hearing the sun god's cries, Indra looked up to see Anjanaya flying toward the sun, his muscles glistening in its sharp rays. For a moment Indra wondered if he ought not simply to be amused by the monkey child's innocence, *but a world in which Suryadeva is threatened*, Indra thought, *is no world at all*. There *is* no life without Surya, and as this world was Indra's domain, he had to protect it at all costs.

So Indra wielded his thunderbolt, the *vajra*, and launched it directly at Anjanaya, striking him right in the jaw just as he opened his mouth wide enough to take a massive bite of the sun. The impact sent the monkey spiraling back through space, through the earth's atmosphere, past the clouds, past the birds, beyond the canopy of trees, and finally crashing with a lifeless thud, unconscious onto the hard earth. In that instant, Anjanaya became Hanuman. (*Hanu* means "jaw," and *man* means "altered" or "disfigured.")

Anjanaya's father, Vayu, came rushing to his son's side. He tenderly scooped up the monkey—who'd shrunk in size as he fell—and held him tightly in his arms. "Who has done this to my child?" he roared, typhoons and tempests gathering at his back. The answer came in the form of silence, so Vayu roared the question again. Still the answer came as nothing but a deafening silence.

As Vayu raged, the air left the earth. The winds immediately ceased. No longer was there a gentle, cooling breeze that gave relief from the midday sun. But no one noticed the burning sensation on their skin, for they had something far more critical to worry about: They could no longer breathe. As the sparse clouds stopped moving above them and hung motionless, suspended in the sky, *all* beings—humans, animals, gods—gasped for air. Doubled over, they looked at each other in bewilderment and horror. Some fell to their knees; others desperately watched their babies as their wild cries turned to silence. No one could speak for lack of air as they sunk to the ground.

In the midst of the suffocating silence, feeble arguments echoed: "But Surya had to survive!" "Anjanaya was too wild!" "Life had gotten out of hand!" "It was unbearable." "What else could Indra have done?"

In desperation, someone, with all the tiny bit of air that was left in their lungs, pleaded to Vayu to return. Vayu promptly reappeared, his unconscious son still in his arms, his eyes swollen and red with weeping. His demand was quieter now, but no less forceful—bring Hanuman back to life or Vayu would depart from this earth forever.

Gasping and desperate to inhale, everyone, including the gods, who had swiftly gathered from every corner of existence, looked at each other. They knew they had a conundrum on their hands. They'd seen how quickly Hanuman's superpowers had grown exponentially over the course of just a few years, and they shuddered at the thought of how those powers would *further* grow as he moved into his impulsive teenage years, and then into adulthood. They all recognized Hanuman's divinity—that was undeniable. But they also worried that if he maintained his thoughtless, reckless, and unruly monkey nature, he'd continue to be a threat to the world.

In a desperate negotiation, the gods offered Vayu a deal. They would bring Hanuman back on one condition: He wouldn't have access to his superpowers unless he was in service to dharma—the highest path, the very core of right action. Then and only then would he be returned as his full self, with access to all his superpowers. Vayu nodded in agreement—anything to feel his son come to life in his arms—as he restored the wind, the breeze rippling through the trees and the relief of oxygen in everyone's lungs.

Lord Brahma, creator of the universe, resurrected the monkey god, who slowly returned to consciousness as the gods, circling around him, whispered their boons. "No weapon will ever be able to harm you again," Brahma whispered first. "From here on out, you will be immune to my thunderbolt," whispered Indra. "And not only to Indra's thunderbolt; you will be immune to *all* fire," whispered Agni, the god of fire. "I give you a hundredth part of my brilliance," blessed a relieved Surya, "to understand and attain all possible knowledge." Boon after boon granted to him, the monkey in Vayu's arms grew in size until the father had to lay his son down on the earth to let him grow fully back into himself.

Upon his revival, Hanuman blinked his eyes open as a new softness spread across his face. He reached out for his father, his movements cautious and controlled, signaling a newfound awareness of his strength. Noticing his perplexity, the gods refrained from explaining the situation, trusting that with the wisdom Surya had granted him, the monkey would soon discover it within himself. They stepped away quietly. The image of father and son, wind and monkey boy, reaching for each other, would stay tenderly seared into their minds for eons.

Life found its rhythm again, as it always does after such crises—the same, but a little different. Hanuman, no longer pulled by the desire for wild antics, steadied himself in service to his fathers. He took up daily practices that included meditation, asanas, and chanting. Sometimes he studied ancient texts, but more often he found the teachings within himself. Out of nowhere, a centuries-old hymn would erupt from his mouth. These eruptions no longer disrupted the ocean tides. Instead, the words wafted over the neighbors' houses, leaving sweet echoes in their hearts.

One day, while in the jungle collecting food for his family, Hanuman encountered Ram, prince of Ayodhya, and his faithful wife, Sita. He was unaware that the man he faced was the very embodiment of Vishnu, the god of preservation, who descends in the form of an avatar to establish balance each time the world is threatened. He did not know that Sita was the daughter of the goddess of the earth, Bhumi, and the living embodiment of purity.

Hanuman was instinctively drawn to their divine presence. As he gazed upon these extraordinary strangers, every drop of wisdom in his body caused him to fall to his knees as his powerful monkey legs collapsed beneath him. Hands raised in reverence, Hanuman swore eternal devotion to Sita and Ram. From that moment on, every word, every thought, every action of his was dedicated to this divine couple, with the name *Ram* riding every breath he took.

From that moment on, Hanuman's loyalty, his unwavering love and devotion, allowed him to accomplish near impossible feats. His service knew no bounds. Whatever Ram needed, Hanuman was there to accomplish, with an open, courageous heart and a steady hand. Prayer beads jangled as, time and time again, he sprang into action. As a prince living in exile in the forest, Ram's needs were many. There were many trials that required the monkey god's help, and for every challenge Ram and Sita encountered, Hanuman was the first to leap to support, uplift, protect, and seek a solution. Through relentless service he further developed his devotion, strength, and clarity. Their life in the forest was rich and filled with a depth of purpose that Hanuman had never known before.

Yet far, far away, a devious plot was being hatched in the minds of the demon king Ravana, who had ten heads and twenty greedy arms, and who, having heard of Sita's exquisite and unparalleled beauty, wanted her for himself. However, Ravana had also heard of Ram's great strength and discipline, so he knew he had to act with caution. Ram was a hunter, and that, Ravana recognized, could be leveraged as a weakness. He ordered his servant Maricha, a *rakshasa* (demon), to disguise himself as a golden deer. As the deer passed them in the forest, Ram and his devoted brother Lakshmana became entranced, for this was a deer unlike any they'd ever seen, and the chase was sure to be electrifying. Lakshmana had drawn a circle in the dust around Sita to protect her while the brothers were hunting. Ravana arrived, disguised as a beggar, and implored her for food and drink. As Sita, with her pure heart, stepped outside the circle to provide sustenance for this stranger, Ravana grabbed her and stole her away to his lair.

Ravana flew for days and days in order to hide Sita as far away from her husband as possible. Meanwhile, the brothers returned to their camp to discover that Sita was missing. Ram's profound grief was felt around the world as he nearly fell into despair, recognizing that it was his own ego that had pulled him away from his beloved, leading to her capture. Once the brothers regained their composure, they learned that it was the evil demon king Ravana who had abducted her.

Ram organized a search party calling upon every man and beast from far and wide. The party searched high and low, west and east and north and south, scouring the lands of this world. After the most exhaustive and thorough search for the demon's kingdom, the party eventually arrived at the edge of the sea, with nothing but miles and miles of blue water ahead of them. A looming sense of defeat overtook the party as they realized that what was between them and the only body of land they had not yet searched—Lanka—was a vast span of water that no one knew how to cross.

As the search party grew silent on the shore, Hanuman turned, walked slowly up a nearby mountain, and sat down. He sat in meditation for days, chanting the name of his guru, who was grieving at the mountain's foot. "Rama, Rama, Rama," the monkey chanted under his breath, and then he chanted it loudly, and then more emphatically, and then as a whisper again. He turned over a ring in his right hand, and then moved it to his left hand, where he fingered it more gently, reverentially.

Days before, Ram had passed purposefully through the ranks of the search party, making his way directly to Hanuman, who welcomed the approaching Ram with his hands pressed together before his heart in *anjali* mudra—a sign of reverence. Pulling a ring from the finger of his right hand, Ram gently took one of Hanuman's monkey hands in his own, dropped the ring into his palm, and closed his fingers around it. "I feel in my heart that *you*, Hanuman, will be the one to find my love. When you find Sita, give her this ring, and she will know that I am close," Ram had said, a note of desperation creeping into his usually calm voice.

For nine days straight Hanuman meditated, gazing toward Lanka. As he chanted Ram's name, his heart swelled as he remembered how his guru's voice broke around Sita's name when he cupped Hanuman's palm in his own. How was it possible for Ram to have such faith in him? Surely his guru wasn't wrong; surely he saw a power in him that he couldn't yet see for himself. Every few hours, as Hanuman sat chanting, a vague feeling erupted in his body—a feeling of lightness, of wind passing beneath him and lifting him up. Hanuman would have described it as the sensation of flying if he knew of his full potential, if his mind was open to what his devotion to dharma had made him capable of. But he was only just on the threshold of this knowing.

While Hanuman stayed immersed in his devotion, the rest of the party, composed of men, monkeys, lions, tigers, bears, and all the other creatures in the wild, huddled at the bottom of the mountain, talking in low tones and debating among themselves. Surely Sita was held captive in Lanka, the only territory they had not covered, which was too far a distance for any of them to jump or fly to, even the strongest among them. But Hanuman was the son of Vayu, the wind god, wasn't he? Surely he possessed his father's speed and strength. After all, they'd *all* heard the story of the monkey child's leap to the sun. If he could jump to such heights, a leap to Lanka should be effortless. So what was Hanuman doing, just sitting there on the mountaintop?

That's when Jambavana, king of the bears, cleared his throat, reminding the party, "You all know the story of little Hanuman's leap to the sun so well, but you forget that he was made unaware of his powers when he was struck in the jaw by Indra. The deal the gods arranged with Vayu was that Hanuman would not have access to his superpowers unless and until he was in service to the dharma. Hanuman has been deeply in service to Ram all these years; he only needs to recognize his powers. We must go to him and help him see, help him remember."

Hours later, Hanuman heard the entire search party approach behind him after their arduous climb up the mountain. "My dear monkey friend," Jambavana began, as he relayed to Hanuman the story of how he had received that great scar, how he'd taken an impossible leap into the sky one day, flying beyond the trees, and then past the birds, and then through the clouds, and then beyond the earth's atmosphere. And as the entire community gathered around, listening intently to Jambavana speak, they saw a hint of remembrance on Hanuman's face as he felt an unfamiliar throbbing, a tingling in his jaw—a remnant of his encounter with Indra.

Jambavana continued talking. He told Hanuman the story of his return to consciousness, of his rebirth. He told him in great detail about each of the boons given to him by each of the gods: his invulnerability to weapons, thunderbolts, and fire. Jambavana spoke until finally the throbbing in Hanuman's jaw grew so strong that a wave of realization washed over him, forcing his whole mouth open, forcing out words he never thought he'd speak, "I am stronger than I ever could have imagined, and I am capable of doing *anything* in service to Rama. My strength, my power, is unlimited."

As Hanuman's acceptance of his true potential resonated in the air, a sigh of relief rippled across the assembled troops. The bear king laughed heartily, shaking his head in joy and relief. The murmurings among the gathering began to grow louder and louder, until they let out a collective gasp as Hanuman rose from his meditation posture, growing solid and vast, and radiating an overwhelming aura of strength and determination.

"He's gonna do it. He's gonna *fly*!" "Hanuman, you've got this!" The whispers turned into chants, echoing across the mountaintop as faith in Hanuman's power united them all. "Hanuman, you've got this! Hanuman, you've got this!" The rallying crew grew in fervor, inspiring Hanuman and bolstering his resolve. In response, Hanuman began to grow larger and larger and larger, his physical form expanding to mirror the vast power that now surged within him. As he expanded, the chants of the party grew louder and louder, their voices harmonizing with his own incantation of "Rama, Rama, Rama."

Hanuman, now as vast as the mountain they stood upon, crouched down on one knee. He looked toward Lanka, so far in the distance that the human eye could not see it. Suddenly, Hanuman felt his feet gathering up the energy of the earth—her strength, her wisdom. He could feel the wind—the father he now remembered—swirl powerfully within him and all around him. He could see Jambavana and all the search party in his periphery, raising their hands and roaring, "You've got this!" And with one final roar of "Ram," Hanuman sprung with a leap that shook the earth to its very core.

He soared skyward, shining a brilliant light reminiscent of the sun. With Ram's ring pressed against his heart, Hanuman traversed the massive expanse of the treacherous sea, facing many tests along the way and even more perilous obstacles upon landing. However, throughout it all, his spirit never wavered. His faith in the mission and the unending support from his community were his guiding forces, continually uplifting him and reminding him of his true nature—that he was powerful beyond imagination, and capable of achieving the seemingly impossible.

MYTH AND MEANING: UNEARTHING OUR SUPERPOWERS

The adventure of Hanuman's leap of faith is but a sliver of the mammoth epic the Ramayana by the great sage Valmiki. The epic tells the rich and complex story of Ram and Sita, the earthly manifestations of Vishnu and Lakshmi—sustenance and grace, the protector of dharma and the embodiment of prosperity. In lifetime after lifetime, Vishnu and Lakshmi meet as new and extraordinary avatars, uniting again and again in the flesh. But in the Ramayana, their relationship in the incarnations of Ram and Sita is complicated by their exile in the forest, and by the fact that Sita spends much of the story imprisoned by the demon king Ravana.

There were many obstacles that presented themselves during Hanuman's flight. These included a shadow-eating demon whom Hanuman allowed to devour him, only to rip through her body and continue flying; and a mountain called Mainaka that emerged from the ocean to serve as a resting place for the monkey, but which Hanuman merely grazed with his hand before flying past so as not to neglect his duty. Upon finding Sita, Hanuman dropped Ram's ring in her lap and whispered words of comfort to her. Hanuman let himself be taken prisoner so he could come face-to-face with Ravana, who set the monkey's tail on fire, not knowing of Hanuman's immunity to fire. Hanuman then shrank to the size of a mouse and gleefully ran through Lanka with his tail afire, leaving the entire demon city in flames. Sita is finally rescued and reunited with her beloved Ram.

But this story is really about Hanuman's leap of faith, his *sraddha*. It's about the power of devotion, the self-trust, and the inner wisdom that it required. It's about the awakening of the dormant superpowers within Hanuman, and how he had to *remember* them in order to take that great leap. It's about the support of the community that helped him discover his inherent potential by reminding him of what was already within him, reminding him of his true nature.

Ultimately this story reminds us of the importance of encouraging each other and witnessing each other, of mutually waking each other up to our dormant inherent dharmic powers that are patiently waiting to be realized and grow to their full potential, so we too can take our own leaps of faith.

The story of Hanuman's early life paints a vivid picture of unchecked desires and a wild, restless monkey mind, characteristics that mirror our own youthful impulsiveness. Like an uncontrolled force of nature, young Hanuman wreaks havoc in his village, just as we often do through our own actions, thoughtlessness, and carelessness.

What I love about this story is that Hanuman's early days are not so much about the consequences of ill will. He simply does what comes naturally to him. The path of destruction he innocently leaves in his wake is the upshot of misdirected energy, much like the potential damage that can come from a teenager driving a car if ruled by their moment-to-moment desires. What's so remarkable about Hanuman is the way he learns to harness that life force after a blow to the jaw—which is ultimately a blow to the ego.

I see this reflected in the ways we chase our unbridled desires, heedless of the damage it may create to ourselves or others. It's often only when we get a similar blow to the jaw—a sobering wake-up call—that we adjust or take stock of our actions and their repercussions. Our careless words and actions toward others in high school are examples of modern-day incarnations of this.

In Hanuman's story, dramatic events unfold to quiet the monkey mind, enabling him to unearth his superpowers and take that great leap of faith. There's the impact of Indra's thunderbolt and the resulting loss of the monkey god's breath. There are years of devoted practice, with an object of devotion Hanuman does not yet know and cannot define, yet fully trusting that he is on his path. There's the meeting, finally, with his guru, his lord Ram, and the renewal of that devotion now that Hanuman knows precisely where to direct it. And then there's the process of self-realization, of remembering *who he is*, which is what ultimately allows him to help reunite what's been severed.

There's something we can take for ourselves from each of these phases of Hanuman's evolution, expanding self-awareness, and discovery of his own superpowers. Ultimately we must remember that our breath, our very life, is our most potent superpower. When we misuse it and throw it away on dramas and worries, clutching on to the past or fearing the future, we unfortunately forget about this most incredible of superpowers—*life*.

In mindfulness practices, we often talk about the monkey mind. If you've ever sat in meditation, or tried to quietly and honestly watch your own mind for more than a minute, whether or not you called it *meditation,* you know very well why the metaphor holds. Our minds are restless, shape-shifting, and volatile. A thought arises, and rather than letting it pass, we chase it—until the next, more compelling thought arises, which we then chase in another direction. It's dizzying.

This flitting about of our minds is innocent enough, and like young Hanuman's, quite natural. But it stifles our clarity about who we really are and what we're up to in this life. What's more, as we saw with Hanuman's irresponsible leap toward the sun, when we get caught in the desire loops of that monkey mind, we forget those we share this world with, and the others on this path who deserve our care, and deserve to be remembered as ones to be held dear. We leap toward our desires many times a day, drawn by voracious hunger for more and misdirected cravings that harm others and deplete nature's resources. Consider, for instance, what our materialism is doing to our own health and well-being and to the Earth's ecosystem; how it contributes to the suffering of so many species.

Had Hanuman succeeded in reaching the sun, the price paid for his satisfaction would've been unimaginably steep: a world without light, which would not have been a world for much longer. In other words, obtaining his desire would have killed him and everyone else on earth. Similarly, while the consequences of chasing after our own cravings may seem less injurious, there are still parts of us that die in the pursuit of anything other than what we have right now. The larger view becomes lost to us. We get pulled from the present moment as we convince ourselves that our identities are somehow tied up in what we lack, in what we long for, in what we will one day have. And then we become lost to ourselves and self-alienated because none of those things have anything to do with who we are at heart.

The discipline and fortitude it takes to still our monkey minds, to direct our attention to what's most healing, most skillful, most uplifting in this life, cannot be underestimated. It takes a hunger and a fixation, but more importantly it also requires a more mindfully chosen point of attention, and this is where the leap to Lanka comes in. As we see later in the story, devotion equates with steadiness.

The Hanuman who fell from the sky was not the same Hanuman who had leapt *into* it. What he bled out as he fell was self-importance. And what hit him, minutes before he hit the ground, was illumination—both literally, in the essence of the thunderbolt, and metaphorically, in his realization that the world is so much bigger than himself.

In the aftermath of Indra's strike and the resulting fall, Hanuman doesn't just lose his self-importance, he also loses (and then recovers) his breath. We speak of Vayu, Hanuman's father and protector, as god of the winds, but he's also the deity of air, space, and breath. The breath is a reminder of the transience of all things. Every breath cycle is a reminder of the cycle of life: the inhalation is creation, the top of the inhalation is the temporary appearance of sustenance, and the exhalation is destruction. To come back to the breath in practice is to be reminded of how careful we must be with what we give our power to.

When Hanuman's breath returns to him, the willingness to squander it on insignificant endeavors is no longer there. Every breath becomes an invitation to turn, again and again, toward his intention.

Breathwork in yoga is the tracing of our attention back repeatedly to present-moment awareness. In doing so, we deepen our connection to the present moment. This is our first superpower: discovering our capacity for devotion—honoring each inhalation by asking what the next moment wants of us, and what we can offer back to it for its gift of life.

Following this transformative event, Hanuman begins his practice with Shiva, the creator of yoga. Shiva teaches him mantras, sun salutations, and fire rituals (*homas*) to harness his energy, and the value of using his energy wisely. Shiva leads him through pranayama, practices of controlling the monkey god's newly significant breath.

Hanuman begins to recognize that his life's dharma is devotion, before he even has a place to direct that devotion. Many of us might resonate with this feeling, sensing a nudge, a call to something deeper, before we even have the words or a sense of direction to know what that call is. Hanuman chants mantras under his breath incessantly, quieting the pleasure-seeking monkey so that the whole of his life becomes a divine song. In that song, there is only trust that this is the path, and that, while it's much more difficult than his boyhood life, it is already infinitely more rewarding.

On one of his daily journeys within the forest, Hanuman runs across Ram, Sita, and Lakshmana. Hanuman immediately falls to his knees before Ram. In that moment, the object of his devotion gets clarified for him; his dharma is resolved, confirmed. Hanuman immediately knows where to direct his devotional efforts. Toward Ram and his beloved Sita.

For us, this may be the moment when we become aware that the practice is working in us, that it is moving us. Something external may happen in our world to validate our having shown up steadily, consistently, for ourselves and our journey to remembering our true nature. It may arrive like a clearer sense of our purpose or a more profound sense of love for all the beings we encounter as we move through our world. It can express itself as a deepened knowing that reenergizes our life.

Hanuman's time in the forest with Sita, Ram, and Lakshmana is one of even deeper disciplined and profound commitment. When he is in service to Sita and Ram, he's utterly certain about the power of these efforts. During this time he feels purposeful and as if he has greater access to his own powers.

When Maricha as a golden deer races past Ram, Ram is compelled by its rarity and elusiveness to chase it. His commitment to Sita and their union momentarily dissipates. He's an example of what we stand to lose when we let ourselves get pulled from our centers in our attempts to chase after the golden things of this world—the things that galvanize our stories of self.

Once Ram, Lakshmana, and Hanuman realize that Sita has been abducted, they gather up a search party and search every inch of land, high and low. This meticulous scouring of the land reflects the moments when we take stock of our inner selves and inquire deeply within. This is the vital journey we take, often in times of crisis, when we go exploring every nook and cranny of our internal landscapes to find a deeper clarity about who we are.

You can perhaps imagine the hopelessness the entire party feels upon reaching the water's edge and looking out into the vast nothingness between India and Lanka, where they'd come to realize Sita was being held captive. Hanuman's powerlessness arises, his sense of having failed his lord twice: first in allowing Sita to be kidnapped, and then again in his inability to recover her. As the party reaches the shore, Hanuman intuitively knows he needs a broader view. Initially it seems strange to the monkeys, bears, and other animals that he would withdraw from the search party at a time when they need his wisdom the most. But Hanuman is compelled to reach the highest point, a remarkable altitude, to get a wider view. And when the altitude isn't enough, he turns inward for the widest view of all. And here's where the work of truly remembering who he is begins.

Hanuman's meditation on the mountaintop reveals more to him than any previous practice had ever revealed. Meditation gives us more than the unglamorous opportunity to confront the errors and delusions of our own stories—the ones that bolster our egos and keep us trapped in limited views, preventing us from opening into the vast field of connectivity. It also helps us remember our expansiveness, our limitlessness, in the face of life's perceived obstacles and apparent constraints.

Meditation brings Hanuman to the threshold of knowing what his devotion to dharma made him capable of. However, it is when Jambavana, the bear king, comes to Hanuman on the mountaintop and recounts his story that Hanuman's true awakening begins. As Jambavana tells the tale of Hanuman's great leap toward the sun, Hanuman starts to truly listen to what he already knew somewhere deep inside.

And this is what *sangha* (community) is for. It's here to reflect what we don't yet see in ourselves, to remind us that we are so much bigger than we think we are, and to support us in moments of forgetfulness. *Sangha* calls us to be our best selves, to walk our highest paths. When Hanuman decides to leap, the soft and excited eyes that meet his and the encouragement in the party's chanting voices remind him that his own powers are beyond even his wildest imaginings. The gestures from the search party reassure him that what his meditation had begun to reveal—that flight was possible—was indeed true. With each iteration of "Hanuman, *you've got this!*" the monkey grows stronger, until eventually he's larger than life.

Sometimes we're lucky enough, or the conditions are right or something else aligns, that we can dissolve our sense of limitation on our own. But as a unifying principle, community often reminds us of the larger, underlying unity—the Sita and Ram beneath all of it. In yoga, the company we keep is of great consequence, as *sangha* will remind us of our true nature when we get lost in the fog, whether it be chasing the golden deer, wreaking negligent havoc in the forest, or being afraid to truly look at ourselves and see what we're capable of. *Sangha* will bear witness to our struggles to remember, and will celebrate our courageous inward journeys to summon our whole, true selves to the present moment. And when we have trouble going inward, they'll go with us to the degree that is possible.

Without community, there would have been no leap of faith for Hanuman. There would have been no reunion of what had been severed. And *this* is what we come together for.

MYTH INTO PRACTICE: STRONGER TOGETHER

Mantra

Om hum hanumate namaha.

Invocation to the god Hanuman. May I be blessed with victory, strength, stamina, and power.

Or:

You've got this.

Meditation

Sit in a comfortable position. Place both hands over your heart, palms facing in, and close your eyes. Scan your body, slowly, from feet to head. Notice the points of contact your body has with both itself and the environment around you: the warmth of your hands over your heart, the way your shirt connects with your skin as your lungs expand and contract, the weight of your thighs against your meditation cushion.

Once your body has fully arrived, turn your attention to the breath. There's nothing to change or manufacture here—though you might find that the breath shifts a bit just by virtue of your giving it attention. Attend to the rising and falling sensations in the stomach and chest, the way your ribs expand to make space for the outside world to enter. Pay attention to the temperature of the inhalation, how it differs from that of the exhalation. Notice the sensations of coolness and warmness in every inhalation–exhalation cycle.

Movement

Move through nine sun salutations, finding those moments when the feet are rooted in the earth, the heart wide open with love and devotion to each breath. Each successive round moves a little bit faster, creating warmth in the body and breath.

Exercise

1. Write down the five things that matter most to you. Then on another page, write down the five things that take most of your time. If the lists are not closely aligned, write down steps you can take today to align these two lists, so that what you value the most lines up with how you spend your actual life energy and moment-to-moment actions.

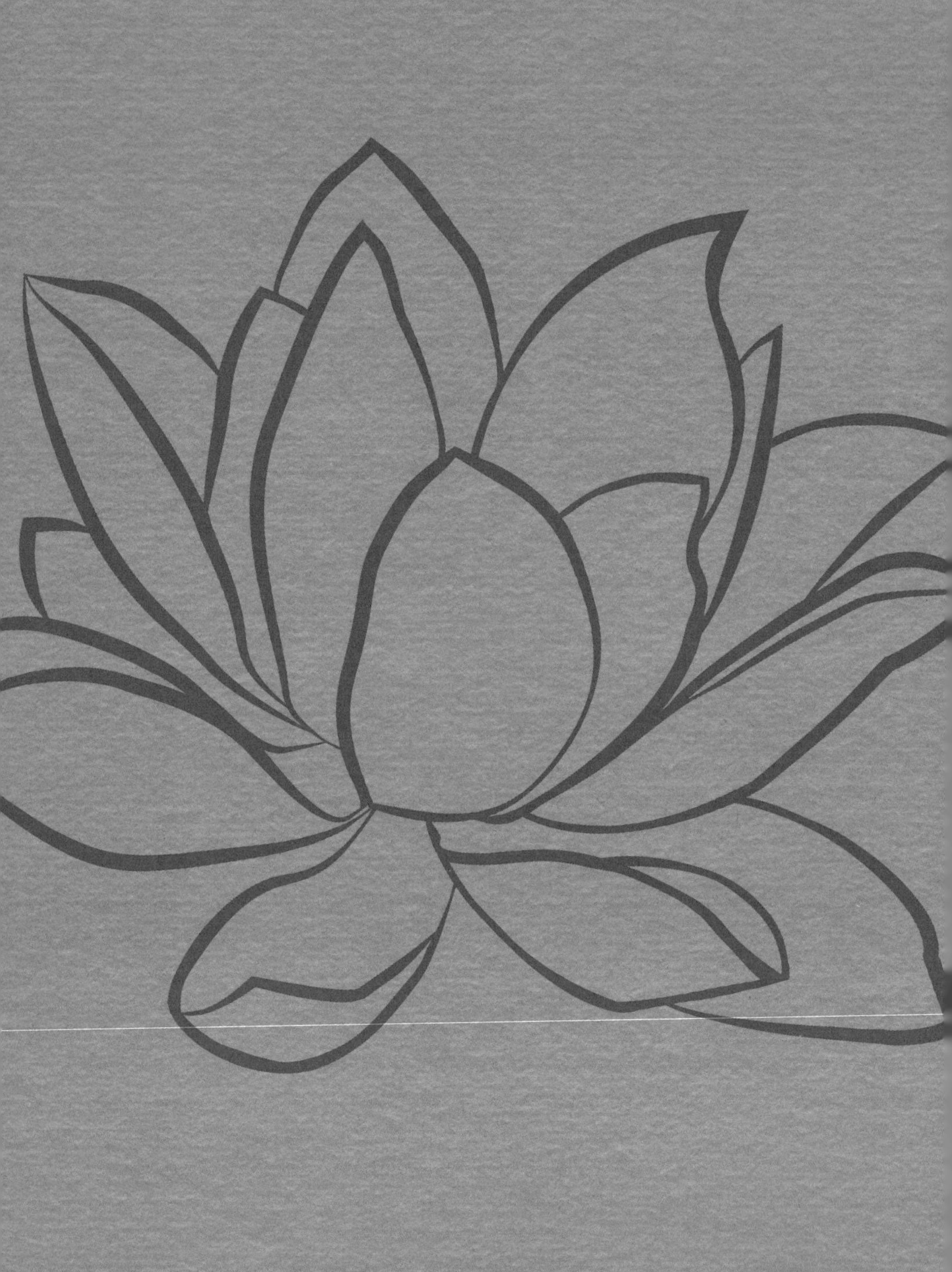

Lakshmi—Garland of Grace

As we voyage back into the infinite folds of time, we stumble upon an old sage named Durvasa, who came into being through Shiva's rage. We flash back to an intense quarrel between Shiva and his wife, Parvati, in which Shiva tipped into a frothing fury and dumped all of his rage into a hapless bystander named Anasuya. This fiery transfer emerged in the form of Anasuya's child, Durvasa, who is known throughout time to be irascible in nature. His name resonated with his character, literally translating to "hard to live with." In his many brushes with gods, devas, and humans alike, the sage often ended up bestowing some horrible curse upon them, and became simultaneously revered and feared during his long life.

Durvasa certainly lashed out in spite; however, more often he harnessed anger as an instrument of change, as a beacon to cut through delusion. Such was his way. His knowledge brought illumination to those who crossed his path, even if through their own suffering from whatever curse he placed on them.

The passage of time did not make the sage less grumpy and agitated. Wandering the earth for eons in service to the awakening and illumination of many, Durvasa had grown rigid and exceptionally harsh. He'd become dispassionate, even in his anger, and every offering became rote and monotonous, his curses lacking their previous flair.

It was then that Durvasa began to contemplate abandoning the earthly realm altogether. He retreated into a deep meditation, sitting for weeks, still, quiet, listening. His brow was furrowed, as usual, and his face tense. Weeks turned into months, until on the one hundred and eighth day he opened his eyes in what he thought was a dream. This dream made every hair on his body stand up, his brow relax, and he almost felt a smile on his face—something that had not occurred in hundreds of years. His heart felt as if it would burst from his chest with a sensation he'd never experienced before—love.

As his eyes came into focus, Durvasa felt an intense sensation of compassion pulsing through him as he took in the most brilliant, effervescent sight of the goddess Lakshmi. The embodiment of abundance, warmth, and grace stood before him, her all-encompassing gaze permeating through to his heart, making him feel full, whole, complete, and even overflowing. Durvasa suddenly wondered if he'd died and this was heaven. Was this divine encounter, this answer to his meditation, his liberation from the cycles of day and night, longing and aversion, birth and death?

The generous arms of the goddess Lakshmi extended toward the sage, offering a garland of such glorious and vibrant beauty that the fragrance of its flowers moved deep into his core and melted him completely. As she draped the radiant garland around Durvasa's scrawny, dusty, wrinkled neck, he felt an awakening that uplifted his whole being. The love, grace, and kindness from Lakshmi's touch flooded his senses, penetrating every cell and transforming him.

As the garland descended around his head, the richness poured through his skull, brain, eyes, ears, nose, and mouth. Every sensory nerve, every cell, felt the bounty of this blessing. The wisdom and grace of all times and spaces washed across him as he looked out upon the world, which came alive in vivid Technicolor. The landscape, which prior to this moment had looked drab, desolate, and without hope, suddenly bloomed with life. This was the boon of Lakshmi, of *sri*, of her elegance and radiance: to suddenly have new eyes to view an old place, and see the stunning beauty of it all.

Imbued with Lakshmi's divine essence, Durvasa closed his eyes and inhaled deeply, reveling in the lingering aromatic bliss. When he opened them Lakshmi was gone, but in her place he saw her exquisiteness reflected everywhere and in everything. The world around him swelled with her pure beauty and elegance. Things Durvasa had never noticed before, ordinary aspects of life, like a fresh bud on the stem, the rhythmic clip-clop of goat hooves, the monkeys frolicking in the tree above, became symbols of vitality and abundance, a feast for his senses.

From this pivotal moment, the sage offered passionate, loving dharma, and everyone flocked to him for his abundant wisdom and generosity of spirit. The world seemed to respond in kind. The sun shone more brightly, the crops were more bountiful, the animals healthier, the flowers more vibrant, and the love and connection between all beings deepened into trust and strength of a community working in harmony. This golden era of benevolence stretched into the annals of time, until no one remembered the once cranky nature of Durvasa's scowl. The earth settled into empathy and compassion as the rule. Love flourished, devotion blossomed, and Durvasa didn't curse anyone. Time seemed to suspend itself in the glory of this peaceful age. Throughout this period, Durvasa was never seen without the garland around his neck and a warm smile on his face.

One day, while Durvasa was in deep meditation, Maha Lakshmi came to him, instructing him to pass the garland of grace on to the next passerby. His first response was complete resistance. This had been the best time of his life of service. It was the greatest gift to be alleviated from the rage of Shiva, to be alleviated from the bitterness, and instead engender smiles and giggles from everyone while walking by. How could he go back to before? However, her voice soothed him through his resistance, and he eventually agreed to hand over the garland to the next person who came his way.

Sitting under a banyan tree alongside a grand path, Durvasa, with soft surrender in his heart, watched a grand procession underway in front of him. This ostentatious procession was the type meant for the more egoic gods and devas.

From the perspective of those in the procession, they saw a dirty, ragged, old, leathery man standing up, removing a wilted, matted, stained, and tired garland from his neck, and walking toward them. No one from the procession recognized him, and they all immediately assumed he was deranged, a look of disgust unknowingly spreading across their faces.

From Durvasa's perspective, he saw the alluring and imposing figure of Indra, riding his elephant, Airavatam, looking toward him with mistrust. With the warmth and grace of Lakshmi still pulsing through him, he ignored the sneers and extended the garland of Lakshmi toward Indra to place upon his glistening neck. A look of horror came across Indra's face and he urged Airavatam to save him from this situation. Without hesitation, Airavatam swung his trunk around, whisked the garland out of Durvasa's hands, and flung it to the earth. He continued to walk on, trampling the garland underfoot, completely unaware of what they had just done.

Stunned, Durvasa stood on the dirt roadside, staring down at the precious garland that had been discarded and stomped on. When he gathered himself, his old rage came flooding back, and he looked after the procession and shouted a curse like no other. He condemned the earth to a life without Lakshmi's grace, a life filled with suffering and darkness. This, he declared, would starve the gods of their devotees, who would be too preoccupied with their own suffering.

The calamitous results of the curse became visible almost immediately. The procession noticed the lushness that had lined their path wilt into brown, dead sticks. Flowers lost color, drooped, and fell off dying stems. When they glanced up, the sun began to fade like it was retreating behind a permanent smog cloud. The crystalline river flowing nearby turned to sludge. Earth's surface went from verdant to parched, cracking under each step of Indra's elephant. Along the path, instead of the acolytes praising this blessed stream of gods and devas, they began to frown and shout obscenities at them.

Seemingly oblivious to the link between the disheveled old man with the crumpled garland and all that was decaying before their very eyes, the devas wore looks of confusion and disbelief. The world seemed to dim with each step they took.

Durvasa's curse rippled out from their footprints to cover the world at large, as smiles turned to mistrust and furrowed brows, abundance in the villages turned into scarcity, neighborliness devolved into fear of one another, crops dried up, waterfalls slowed to a trickle, and the community's natural balance with nature turned into a muttering of "What can I take?" It was a complete dimming of the spark of life across the world.

The garland lay crushed into the cracked earth as the sage skulked away into the shadows, grieving for the choice the world had made: to turn away from the beauty, generosity, empathy, and creativity, and instead to descend into greed, fear, and mistrust.

Years went by, then decades, then centuries. Sometimes the grandmas and aunties would tell young ones the lore of a time long ago full of joy, warmth, and love. During this period it wasn't just the earth and her creatures that suffered; even the gods suffered, as no one paid any attention to them anymore. Neglected and ignored, they soon began to lose their power. After all, it is the power of love, adoration, and devotion that gives them their divine strength.

Durvasa washed his hands of the chaos, while the gods stressed and grumbled about what had unfolded due to Indra's pompous and callus act. That single moment cost the world the grace of Lakshmi—the grace of kindness, joy, appreciation, and awe. They realized it when the folks stopped acknowledging the incredible gift that was each moment of life and the divinity of nature. Lakshmi didn't make a big thing of it; no war, drama, or argument. She simply retreated and let humans sit in the shadow and sense of her absence.

They knew they had to find her. The only one who knew where she was was her consort, her other half, Vishnu.

The gods pleaded with Vishnu to draw her back to the surface, to give the humans another chance. At first Vishnu had ignored their pleas, but finally, due to his own desire to reunite with his beloved, he rose up and embarked on a journey to their sanctuary, to which he knew Lakshmi had retreated.

Lakshmi and Vishnu had spent many millennia floating together on the milky ocean of consciousness, and this was their go-to spot. Everyone was tremendously anxious and excited for her return, so they followed Vishnu to the edge of this vast body of water. However, upon their arrival, they found the asuras (demons) already immersed in the water, attempting to bring Lakshmi to the surface. They'd been eavesdropping on the gods, waiting to find out where she was, and had rushed to the scene to lay claim to the goddess of wealth and prosperity before Vishnu arrived. The prospect of possessing the elixir of abundance was just too enticing for them to ignore.

Greedily, they churned at the ocean, but to no avail. Despite their best efforts, they got nothing. Just swirly water. The gods and devas watched in amusement, knowing that Lakshmi would never ascend for such shadowy brutes. Exhausted and defeated, the asuras retreated to the ocean banks in a puddle.

It was then that Vishnu turned himself into the longest *danda* (staff) in history and plunged into the seemingly bottomless ocean until he hit the solid surface deep below. The gods and devas aligned themselves on either side of the staff and began to churn. They churned night and day with the force of the entire universe. They churned for all sentient beings, for the return of praise from their subjects, for grace and beauty itself. They gave it every last drop of energy they had. To their surprise and consternation, nothing happened. All they had was just more swirling water.

Meanwhile the demons, a bit rested, started to notice that the gods were failing and began to gain energy from this failure, as any good demons do.

Vishnu remained a solid *danda* in the waters of his beloved, while the gods and devas returned to the surface, wiped out. As they broke through the surface of the water, they could see the asuras gaining energy, and brokered a deal with them: If the asuras joined the efforts to churn, they too would benefit from the blessings of Lakshmi's return. As was standard among the beasts, they began a vicious infighting that resulted in curses, bloodshed, and egos being crushed; however, they finally agreed and joined the gods on the staff, and so began the fierce and seemingly endless task of churning—asuras at the base and devas on the top. No one could have guessed what happened next.

As the combined efforts of the gods and asuras churned the ocean, what surfaced was not Lakshmi and her *amrita*, but the most noxious poison known throughout time—the *halahala,* also known as *kalakuta.* This antithesis of *amrita* could decimate anything it came in contact with. Panic spread among the gods and asuras.

As the inky poison began to spread across the surface of the water, Indra knew he had to take action. It was his fault, after all, that they were all there searching for Lakshmi. It was his ego and presumptuousness that had caused him to disregard her gifts. He leapt to Mount Kailash to find Lord Shiva and bring him to the water, as he was the only one who would know what to do in this moment that had the potential to end all of time as they knew it.

After some resistance, Shiva was intrigued enough with this circus. He arrived on the scene, and seeing this noxious poison spreading far and wide, he simply leaned over, placed his lips on the surface of the water, and slurped up every last drop of the poisonous *halahala*. As he drew it all in, he held it in his throat, earning him the name Neelkantha, the blue-throated one. Everyone watched in utter awe as Shiva then began to chant and chant and chant. This chanting boomed through all space and time, awakening all that had fallen into a sleep, into a state of forgetting, as they instantly joined the vibration. In this mantra, Shiva transmuted the poison into power, the power to wake up, to join life and use pain and poison as another potent force of energy.

With the *halahala* no longer a threat, the demons and devas returned to churning, this time without any expectations. This time they simply focused on the churning itself and not the potential boon of Lakshmi's return. Suddenly they noticed a rush from below, a rush of pure glory rising to the surface.

In that moment the drabness that had become normalized turned into near Technicolor. From the aquamarine of the water to the brilliant blue of the sky, the warm golden light of the sun to the vibrant colors of the sea and land, the world around them seemed to awaken and burst with colors that had disappeared for as long as they could remember.

Sensing her return in his every cell, Vishnu awaited his beloved as those around gasped in excitement and awe. Breaking through the surface of the water, Lakshmi floated upon a vast kaleidoscopic lotus with her elephant guards showering her with water on either side. She was adorned in the rich color of red, hair gleaming, face brilliant. Her right hand was in *abhaya* mudra, the gesture of pure fearlessness, and the left hand was near her left hip, open and pouring out gold and offerings of inexhaustible prosperity. This gesture was not for greed and money; it was to signify that she was always giving of her richness of life and prosperity, her endless bounty, and her promise for abundance of breath.

MYTH AND MEANING: ENOUGHNESS

The layered messages of this purana profoundly echo the transformative power of perspective. Ultimately we are responsible for the way in which we experience the world around us, molding our experiences through our perceptions. The question is, do we spend most of our time looking toward all that is lacking and not enough? Or do we engage with the divine energy of Lakshmi, embracing the abundance of each breath, the warmth of the sun, the breath in our body, the love we receive, the ocean waves, the human connection, community, and the natural world?

Each moment gives us the opportunity to wear the garland and experience the vibrancy of life in its rich tapestry of living moment to moment with eyes of wonder. The practices of yoga guide us toward this sense of awe, toward fostering an acute awareness of the breath-to-breath gift of it all.

We enter the story with a conundrum for the Western mind: rage as a sage? This notion is a reminder that rage can create power and energy, a force that has a place in the world for both healing and awakening. Anger, perhaps more than any other emotion, moves us to change. However, if not melted into the fluidity, into the watery essence of life, anger leaves the one who harbors it dehydrated and burnt out. Even the wisdom of a sage, born from rage and capable of lighting a fire for both god and mankind, eventually succumbs to exhaustion and ends up tired, bedraggled, and devoid of power, feeble in its force.

In the story, the opportunity to shift arrives in the form of Lakshmi and the garland, which represents the grace of each breath. The transformative moment is simple and instantaneous—much like my experience of paying attention to the stunning power of life. The moment I lift my head up from the mental spin of not-enoughness, of my perceived scarcity, is the moment I can feel the abundant grace of life. It's a shift as simple as a change in perspective, a redirection of attention, a brief suspension of judgment.

This pivot is a testament to the fact that the human mind often tends to overcomplicate everything. We imagine that it will take endless amounts of time, money, and energy to find happiness, to experience beauty, when it's quite simply and always available, waiting to be noticed amid the clatter and clamor of our everyday lives. We endlessly focus on the future with a when-this-then-that caveat, often overlooking the abundant joy and beauty present in our lives right now.

Durvasa meditates to receive the answer to his discomfort of this human world. This is a potent reminder that we too can turn to meditation in our quest for clarity and peace. Our own meditation can be formal—seated, candlelit, as part of our routine—or it can simply be a momentary pause, a reflection on all that is. Through these moments of quiet introspection, we learn to appreciate the simple, everyday miracles that we often overlook. Like Durvasa, we too will start to see beauty in the ordinary aspects of life. We too will see life in Technicolor: the breathtaking colors of the sunset sky, the quiet comfort of a warm cup of tea, or the sincere smile from a stranger. It is here, in these beautifully ordinary moments, that we can learn to recognize and celebrate the grace of life and abundance, the grace of Lakshmi. This is where grace lives.

We witness the divine grace sink into Durvasa, transcending his physical boundaries and spreading outward like ripples.

It doesn't just fill him, it permeates in all directions, leaving an indelible mark on everyone in its wake. The transformation isn't just confined to his individual experience; it becomes a shared phenomenon that resonates on a communal level, awakening dormant grace within those who bear witness. This represents that ripple effect we often witness, when a simple act of smiling triggers an inner shift that's palpable and swift within someone else, often inciting a reciprocal smile. This cascading effect illuminates the interconnectedness of our experiences and how we can, like Durvasa, become conduits of grace.

The garland as a whole, and each delicate and fragrant flower within it, conveys an endless flow of life that links all living forms and the preciousness of it all. From the moment this garland lands on the crusty sage, he finds himself emanating an aura of radiance, illumination, and optimism. Connectedness has that power. When we feel as if we're linked to all living things from the past, present, and future, our vitality becomes palpable. The garland invokes the cyclical process of feeling separate and returning to interconnectedness.

However, the normalization of fear, mistrust, and greed brings us deeper into our shadows rather than drawing us closer to grace. At every moment, with every interaction, we have a choice to look toward what is beautiful, full, and enough, or toward that which is lacking, ugly, and empty. What will we choose?

Even as the garland fades, it continues to symbolize the power of finding beauty in all things that express life. It's the beauty-is-in-the-eye-of-the-beholder story played out.

Following the arc of Durvasa's transformation from vengeful to benevolent, we witness how his inner experience reflected outwardly, making him appear more radiant and alive to the outer world as well. This is analogous to an app's filter option on today's electronic devices. By just selecting a filter, you and the world around you can take on an artificial glow (at least as seen through our tiny screens). However, the sage achieves this through the boon of Lakshmi. It works both ways: He sees the world, and the world sees him, as if through one of those modern-day filters.

When he receives the message from Lakshmi that it's time to pass on the elixir, Durvasa initially hesitates, but he doesn't expend too much time or energy on resistance. He's living through the lens of trust, which allows him to feel the grace of her offering without the attachment. This nonattachment relates to so much in life, but it's a particularly potent concept to consider with respect to love. When we're asked to let a particular form of love go, it is as if we suddenly lose all of what it was, as if its essence must be discarded. However, this transition could actually encourage the love to grow—we don't need the physical presence to feel the love. Love isn't all an illusion just because it had an expiration date. Once we know love, we can never *unknow* it.

The moment the sage opens his eyes and sees the procession with Indra mounted on his powerful elephant, he's filled with clarity and resolve. Without grasping or second-guessing, he rises up and removes the garland from his stained neck, and reaches his arms high with his offering. Here again I return to the smiling-at-someone metaphor. Have you ever felt gross, like you haven't showered or pulled yourself together, or you have acne, or you're worried you have food in your teeth? At those times we feel closed off and separate from the world around us; we see ourselves through the lens of "What do I look like?" or "How is the world judging me?" We shut down, drop our heads, don't engage, and become detached. But while Durvasa wears the garland, he doesn't notice his appearance at all. He's engaged, his smile is bright, his arms are open. This sums up the Lakshmi energy. When we're not judging or criticizing ourselves (and therefore others), we become receptive to the beauty of life and connection.

Durvasa acts from this space as he reaches up to offer the garland, and in response he encounters the disdain on Indra's face. This doesn't bother Durvasa, because he makes his offering from a space of abundance and grace.

However, the moment Indra rejects the garland and Airavatam the elephant, literally and figuratively, tramples upon it, is the exact moment that *sri* (grace) and Lakshmi retreat. In the story, the sage spews the curse. However, Lakshmi had already begun to retreat into the vast ocean of consciousness, away from human disregard for the precious-ness of every living thing, interaction, and breath. When she's forsaken, she doesn't put up a fight, like Durga does, or decap-itate someone, like Kali does; she simply departs. It's like that moment of being on some mountain peak, taking in a most beautiful sunset, and suddenly finding all that is wrong with the moment: the cold, what someone you're with just said, what happened earlier that is still running through your mind. In a heartbeat, the moment's beauty is lost. No one fights you, or invites you to come back to presence and awe. You're simply left there with your sense of lacking.

In the story, Indra's judgment initiates Lakshmi's depar-ture. Something so sacred and beautiful was happening, but Indra assumed that something potent would only come in a certain form: It would look radiant, effulgent. When Durvasa reaches up with dirty hands offering the bedraggled garland of flowers, Indra dismisses it. He not only overlooks the grace, he tramples upon it. Our assumptions, expectations, precon-ceived notions, and narrow ideas of how something should be can lead us to miss what *does* show up and the *way* it shows up. We overlook beauty in unexpected forms, in what appears ugly—the murky, muddy waters that give rise to the lotus, the decomposing organic matter that gives birth to new life, the dark thunderclouds that quench the dry earth.

When the gods arrive on the scene to encourage Lakshmi's return, they notice the asuras attempting to capture Lakshmi.

The demons desire to control her and gather the elixir for their own greedy purposes. When the demons fail, the gods confidently get to it, assuming that she'll return immediately in response to their efforts. However, they too are unsuccessful. The gods are stunned, as they have never failed before.

The gods balk when they hear the murmurs of those gathered suggesting they work together with the asuras. However, they eventually see the necessity. This symbolizes bringing our own shadow forces and light forces together to draw forth riches deeper than any single part of us can reach. It is the friction of this moment that creates action. "High vibes only" is not a part of the teachings of yoga; instead, we're called to know the shadows, to walk through the muck, to gain a wider view.

As both the gods and asuras—light and shadow forces—begin their collaborative churning, they each have to put aside their differences, working in symbiosis with all the other parts to accomplish the task at hand. Our darker thoughts or more reactive tendencies can lead us to deeper self-understanding and growth, if we dare to examine them. Much like the different systems in our body, our light and shadow forces need to work together, to churn together, not in an effort to eliminate the other, but to bring forth a greater depth of richness and understanding from within ourselves. Just as our body works in harmony to keep us alive, so too must our inner forces find a way to coexist, for it's in the balance that our true self resides.

But as the gods and asuras churn together, they expect that with their joint efforts this time they will manage to extract Lakshmi from the ocean. This is where I always get caught. I'm always so sure that this effort, this coming together, will produce the desired results. Ha! The clarity here feels so relevant. As Krishna says to Arjuna in the Bhagavad Gita, "You have the right to your efforts, your actions, but not the outcome" (chapter 2, verse 47).

Instead of the desired result—Lakshmi's return—what comes to the surface is the most noxious poison. It's all the things we've stuffed down deep inside ourselves, even the things our ancestors stuffed down. This is why practicing yoga comes with a warning label: Don't go any further unless you're ready to have all your hidden poisons come to the surface. If we don't include all of ourselves in the process of living, then we will never reach the elixir. The practice of yoga begins when the toxic parts that subtly or not so subtly steer our life are brought to the surface and healed and integrated.

Shiva, the representation of creation and destruction, the symbol of transformation, most often the part of life that is the surrender of self, of body, shows up on the scene to slurp up a poison that every other aspect of life wants to run from. Shiva walks toward the *halahala* with no hesitation and takes it in, not fearing death.

He uses his power and attention to transmute poison into potent energy through mantra. This represents the repetitive mental patterns—our tapes that keep playing over and over in ways that permeate every living moment. Practice provides us with the tools and inner resolve to transform our inner poisons into our strengths. Once we have discovered how to transmute poison into power, we are liberated from the need to quell our shadow parts, to hide our wounded parts. Instead, they are welcomed in and woven into the multicolored, textured tapestry of our lives.

We can't overlook mantra as a powerful tool, one that has a place in so many traditions, cultures, and ages. It has the power to direct the mind toward a focal point, to cease the chasing, the endless churning of thoughts until one believes they are crazy. We have the power to change the poison of our thoughts through focused mantra, a conscious repetition that retrains the mind.

The eventual ascendance of Lakshmi is less important in my interpretation of this purana. It suggests finality or some reward in the most obvious of ways. However, for me, her return embodies the effort to use all of ourselves—good and evil—to clear our viewfinder and see the preciousness in every living aspect of life. All sense of lacking or not-enoughness fades, scarcity and inadequacy fades, and we experience the resplendent nature of life through the deep sense of enough-ness of abundance and grace, a deep sense of Lakshmi.

MYTH INTO PRACTICE: RECEIVING ABUNDANCE

Mantra

Om namo Lakshmi.

Salutations to the goddess Lakshmi, ripe with abundance, prosperity, grace.

Or:

I am enough. I have enough. I give enough.

I get enough.

I am enough.

Meditation

Imagine floating in a seated position on the still waters of a pond. Allow the stem of your spine to root into the earth, the stem descending through the water into the rich nutrients of the mud. From that nourishment, the stem of the spine grows taller toward the light and rises through the crown of the head. Soften the shoulders as your being rests in its innate power.

Notice the feeling of the heart rising, opening like the petals of a lotus flower, and ascending through the mind and out the crown of the head. Sit in openness, from the strength of the root, through the vitality of the stem to the fragrant, colorful blossom at the heart. Begin to bring attention to the flow of breath in and out, like waves on the shore, coming and going—a complete naturalness in its fluidity.

Movement

Come to a standing position. Imagine the deep roots of the lotus flower still connected to the earth below. Sense this connection to the ground, and from there, stack your body into a graceful, strong alignment.

From this grounding, begin to move your body intuitively, feeling a sense of floating or moving through water. You can play music if that supports you. In your movements, notice the way one part of your body ripples into other parts. Start to move in all directions, perhaps lifting your feet. Imagine seaweed floating in the ocean, and how it can move dynamically in all directions: forward, back, side to side, and twisting. Allow your body to move in all these planes of motion.

Try to sustain this fluid, intuitive movement for as long as you can. As you begin to wind down, do so slowly, making the motion gradually slower and smaller until you return to stillness. You might feel a sense that you are still moving, ever so subtly.

Exercise

1. Grab some paper and make two columns, one labeled "Enough" and the other "Lack." In the Enough column, write all that you feel is sufficient and grace-filled in your life, and in the Lack column, write what you feel is lacking or not enough. Notice which column is easier to fill up. Keep bringing attention toward the ENOUGH column.

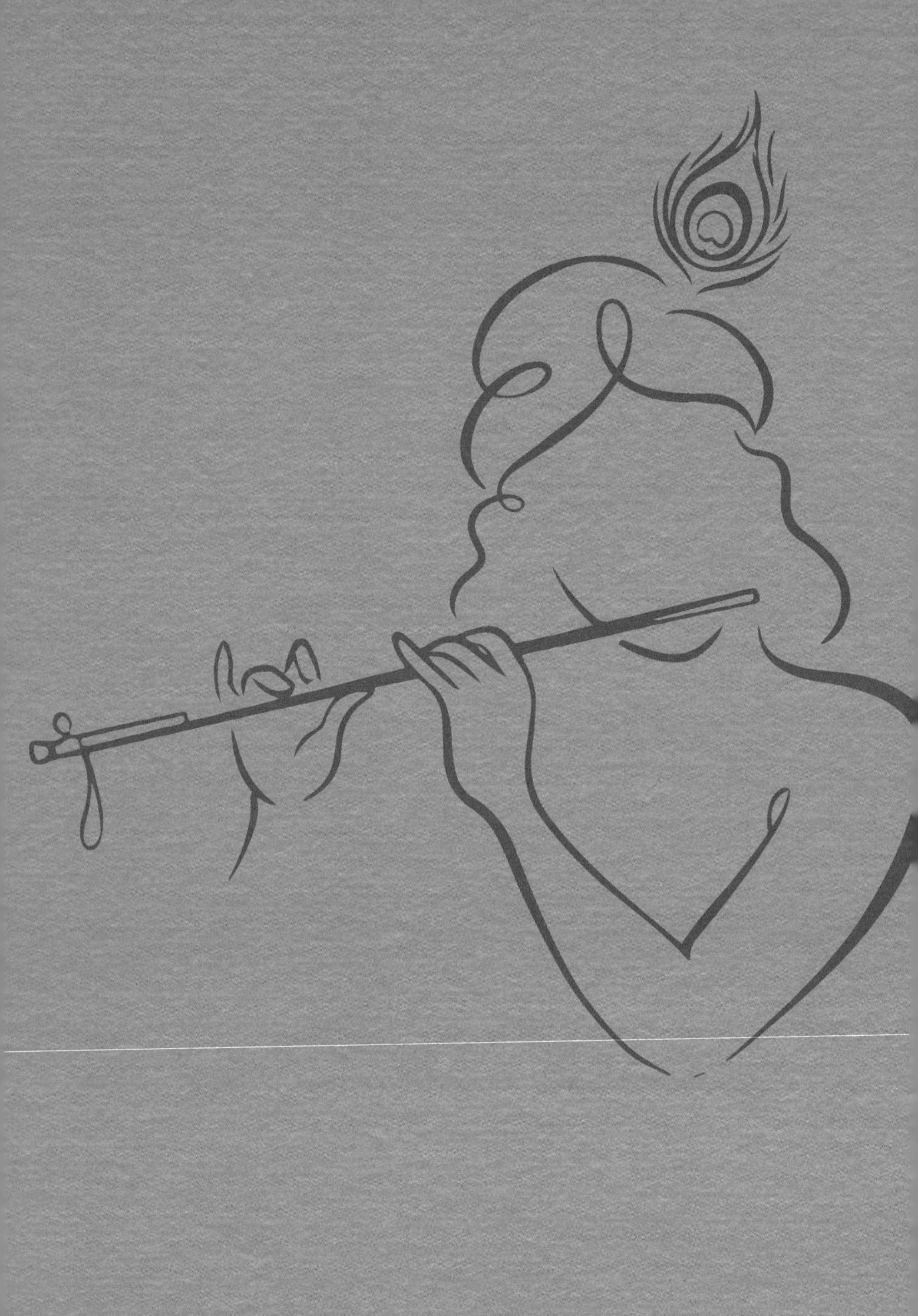

Rasa Lila—The Divine Play

*R*asa can be translated as "nectar" or "divine," and *lila* means "play" or "dance." Let us enter the divine play.

We find ourselves unfurling into this epoch shrouded in time's mists, when we find King Vasudeva and his queen, Devaki, imprisoned by the queen's evil tyrant cousin Kansa. Consumed by their greed and desire to gorge on every last drop of the earth's bounties, Kansa and his friends destroyed the planet, draping themselves in jewels at the expense of the suffering of all others.

During one of his marauding quests, Kansa came across an oracle who told him that his doom would come at the hands of a son born from his cousin and her husband, the king. This chilling omen sparked the flame of paranoia within Kansa, who, taking no chances, constructed elaborate and false accusations to have the queen and king imprisoned within the cold stone walls of a dungeon.

The kingdom that was once ruled with fairness and compassion spiraled into chaos, deception, fear, mistrust, and suffering. But even though they now lived in treacherous conditions as prisoners, the king and queen's joy and love for each other could not be quelled. This love expressed itself in the form of a child, whom Kansa, fearing the prophecy, promptly murdered. Devaki and Vasudeva's love continued producing children, and Kansa ripped each one of them from their arms, exterminating them. His fear of his own death was now his every thought, and it consumed him with more paranoia and rage than before.

Nonetheless, love kept persevering, and though the lives born of this love ended tragically, they represented the undying union and trust between the king and queen. Even in the face of constant tragedy and loss, they persisted and had another son. This time they planned to sneak the newborn out of prison, a feat they managed to accomplish with the help of loyalists. The young offspring was placed in a canoe on the great river, and eventually landed downriver in a remote village of cowherders.

This infant was Krishna. The details of his arrival soon blurred with time, as he was lovingly raised as the son of humble cowherders Nanda and Yashoda. However, his unique aura was undeniable, setting him apart from his peers, with the most striking of all features—a divine blue complexion.

Krishna grew up to become the most alluring, beloved, playful, joyful heartbreaker. He played the flute, which made all the women swoon. The *gopis* (female cowherders) spoke of him continuously and passionately. They were captivated and drawn toward him like moths to a flame—and what a brilliant flame he was!

Despite all of this attention, Krishna remained steady in his devotion and practices, caring for his adoptive parents and herding the village cows with unwavering diligence.

One late afternoon, as the golden hues of the fading sun dimmed in the twilight, Krishna made his way to his favorite clearing in the forest. Enclosed within an emerald circle of trees, a vast glade basked in the luminous light of the moon, emerging from the receding veil of daylight. Leaning against a mighty tree, Krishna pulled out his flute and began playing melodies that wafted through the forest, as if the heavens had come to earth. So immersed was he in this conversation with the infinite spirit that all of his mundane human concerns dissolved into insignificance.

Meanwhile the *gopis* busied themselves in the rhythm of their daily lives, performing their duties: milking the cows, cleaning the stables, tending the children, washing the dishes, cleaning the homes, fetching the water, and chopping the wood.

As they went about their tasks, a soft, alluring melody in the distance began to permeate the air, a sound they felt more than heard. The enchanting notes infiltrated their lives, and as their hearts surged and beat a bit harder, their legs became weak and an intoxicating dizziness invaded their activities. The ethereal sound grew, and with it grew their distraction from the tasks at hand. Every attempt to stay focused was met with bewilderment, as each one felt this overwhelming call. Beyond reason, each *gopi* experienced a pull so fierce, so compelling, it felt as if they were being drawn out to the ocean in a rip current, and no amount of paddling could stop the force.

Before they knew it, all of the women were overwhelmed by the pull of this breathtaking sound. The woman milking the cow stood up and distractedly tripped over the bucket, spilling milk everywhere as the cow looked back to see what the ruckus was. The woman cleaning the stables dropped the pitchfork and stepped in cow manure on her way out the door. The woman tending the children set them down with her mother and stumbled toward the forest. The woman washing dishes dropped them midway, shards of crockery left shattered in the sink, as she drifted nearly in a trance toward the call. The woman cleaning the floor abandoned her mop; the woman fetching water dropped her bucket; the woman chopping wood threw the ax; and they all began to run toward this enticing symphony, this divine call. Through the fields, over rivers, through the forests, they trudged with hearts on fire, an unquenchable thirst in their longing.

After what seemed like a hundred years trekking through the dense forest, the *gopis* broke into a clearing and found themselves in a massive circular opening. This heavenly *vraja* was a celestial haven, a mystical place filled with other-worldly beauty, floral scents, and river breezes. The *gopis*, who numbered 1,008, gasped as they halted in pure awe. Looking around, they absorbed this divine spectacle of a ring of trees around the clearing that was lit up with the fullness of the moon hanging above them. From the astonishment of this perfect circular clearing and the radiant moon and stars above, from the soft touch of the night upon their skin and the sweet, intoxicating smell in the air, they each turned their attention back to the luscious sound that had lured them there in the first place. Each one of their senses was overpowered, and as their eyes dropped from the radiant moon, they noticed the gleaming light from where the captivating sound was emanating. When their eyes finally landed upon the effulgent light surrounding Krishna, they were nearly robbed of their breath. There he was, the most alluring delight, the most resplendent glory that is Krishna.

As 1,008 sets of eyes landed upon him, Krishna's love blossomed in equal volume. In this sublime moment it became abundantly clear that each *gopi* saw only Krishna. They were utterly oblivious to the presence of the others, their eyes singularly focused on the astounding sight of Krishna in all his glory. Their eyes only saw the pure essence of his love.

Every *gopi* had been pulled from her daily duties and responsibilities, pulled by this divine call that had bypassed logic and penetrated the heart. Unaware of the others, each heart was tuned to the creator of that celestial call. The creator of love. The creator of passion and pure divinity.

Krishna, swollen with this piercing love of devotion and the hearts of all those who had abandoned the norm to attend to the call of the heart, seemed to become grander than ever. As his eyes met the entranced *gopis*, a gentle smile curved up on the right side of his mouth, sending a ripple of swooning among the ring of women. Detaching from the tree, he multiplied into 1,008 forms of himself, of love and the heart, appearing individually before each one of them.

Thus began the dance of Krishna and the 1,008 *gopis*, as they swayed to the music, the rhythm wrapping each pair into a bubble of lyrical flow. Time seemed to stand still as the movement began to rise and fall, slow and then speed up, each participant suspended in pure, unadulterated freedom.

All of the woodland creatures, from the deer to the birds, paused from their busyness as they were drawn into the great dance that was before them. The stars above shone brighter and the moon nearly took on the vibrancy of the sun, as the sun's luminous rays bounced off the moon's surface and beamed down sparkly light into the perfectly synchronized frolic.

Looking down from a bird's-eye view, there was a precise circle with 1,008 *gopis* each dancing with one of the 1,008 Krishnas, not one of them noticing the other. As the rhythm surged in its intensity, a swell of notes building upon each other, the movements—spinning, dipping, lifting, swaying, leaping—all matched it in perfect concert, in perfect unison with Krishna, the harmony of each being aligned perfectly as they were all carried to what appeared to be the buildup toward the apex, the great climax of the dance.

The mounting intensity escalated within the immense circle, as the *gopis* lost themselves in the *lila,* simultaneously finding an inner depth, discovering a part of themselves that had never been revealed before. The intensity of their movement—their breath, their dresses whirling this way and that, the glistening sweat upon their skin, and above all the ecstasy on their faces—told a tale of profound transformation.

Approaching the summit of the fervor, women swirled with their eyes tightly closed, spinning at dizzying speeds, feet pounding the ground causing tremors across the land, and arms floating and flying in all directions. As the dance hit its apex, an audible murmur began to permeate the air, sounding like the rumbling of a far-off stampede. This rumble grew louder with each passing moment, until faint whispers of "He's mine, he's mine, he's mine" could be heard. These whispers then grew to clear sounds, then louder and louder and louder, until the deafening declaration, *"He's mine, he's mine, he's mine!"* resonated with such force that it reverberated in their chests. Their hands clenched into fists, their bodies became tense with anticipation.

In this heightened moment, 1,007 of the *gopis* opened their eyes, hoping to look directly into their beloved's eyes, hoping to see Krishna, hoping to affirm that he was theirs and theirs alone. However, in that instant he vanished. Disappeared.

Confused and stunned, they each found themselves amid 1,006 other *gopis* in a similar situation, all with clenched fists and wild looks in their eyes, and bodies covered in sweat. *Who are all of these people? When did they get here? Where is my Krishna?* These questions, asked of no one in particular, buzzed around them as they wandered aimlessly. With no answers in sight, they slowly wandered back to their respective homes, chores, duties, and responsibilities. They were left utterly dumbfounded. *Did this really happen? Was it all a dream? Where did he go?* Each one had been so certain that Krishna belonged to them. They had begun planning their future with him—houses and children and vacations to the countryside. But now they found themselves empty-handed, befuddled, and exhausted, and yet strangely enlivened at the same time.

Meanwhile, back in the nearly empty circle, one dance continued. One *gopi*, Radha, kept her hands open, palms to the sky, eyes open, and heart boundless to the oneness of her and the real Krishna. Completely immersed in the dance, the play, the *rasa lila*, she allowed the flow of love to pour through her, never once trying to hold it, grasp it, own it, or preserve it. It was free. Free to flow, come and go, rise and fall, expand and contract. She never once tried to possess the feeling, the experience, or Krishna. This complete abandonment of self and attachment to her beloved allowed the dance to continue—the union of two becoming one.

And so it is said that even today Radha and Krishna continue this dance, the dance of complete immersion in the moment, in love, in the heart, in the *rasa lila*.

MYTH AND MEANING: LET GO AND DANCE

Rasa or *ras* can be translated as "sap," "juice," "essence," "taste," or "flavors." It's what brings forth the power of emotion when you hear that song, see that painting, or feel that dance in your own body. The human expression of emotion is a powerful force, and in that moment we witness this overwhelming emotion, this swell of feelings that overtakes logic and has the *gopis* swirling in complete *ananda* (bliss).

Ras means the divine flavors or the ambrosia of life. *Lila* translates as "divine play." It is the reminder that we are all a spontaneous expression of the absolute. We're all here to express, play, and act out art through this body, this breath, this life. We're all acting out characters in this grand play, each with unique traits, ideas, beliefs, and aspirations. The dance of Krishna and the *gopis*, each with their unique interpretation of joy and devotion, beautifully captures this concept of *lila*.

So here we are exploring the divine play. Somehow we arrived in the body, in this moment in time, and have become the character in the mysterious story unfolding through our moment-to-moment experiences. We look behind the theater curtain at the inner workings and then we join the dance of this life wholeheartedly. Let's play.

We find this love, desire, play, delight, abandon, dance, and full participation in the practices of bhakti yoga, the yoga of the heart. The Bhagavata Purana is noted as one of the seed text for the bhakti movement, which was a social and spiritual movement that allowed practitioners to have a personal relationship with the divine in its many forms. Prior to this movement, only priests and specific castes could access the teachings and then disseminate them to a *sadhaka* (student).

This movement was revolutionary in the way it opened up the possibility for the student to connect directly with the divine and to access the divine within themselves. This was radical and considered subversive.

Krishna's many stories often speak of this intimate relationship one could have with the god within and without. In the Bhagavad Gita, Krishna poses as a chariot driver to Arjuna, who is in a critical moment in his life. Krishna says to Arjuna, "Enter yourself, the gates of oneness, through me." This theme of a direct, intimate relationship became fodder for poets such as Rumi, Kabir, and so many more, and remains a central tenet for many spiritual paths today.

The *rasa lila* (or Krishna tandava) embodies the divine play or divine dance and is the perfect display of formless love. It places us in the ordinary world of all the *gopis* who represent the embodiment of spirit manifest through its myriad expressions. We find them performing regular life tasks—the duties and daily activities we agree to while in a body. We witness how each *gopi* begins to feel the call to the heart, the call to know more, to go deeper, to explore more than the chores of society. We watch how the call gets louder and louder, until the rational mind—the one that tells us to stay in our lane, to follow the rules we didn't even participate in setting—is overcome by the allure of Krishna's flute.

Much like the *gopis*, we too live by a set of rules we didn't create and norms we didn't agree to consciously. Most of those norms separate us from ourselves, our deeper wisdom, and from one another and the natural world. Through these social conventions, we're also often cut off from the One, the force that connects us all into the whole of life, living and breathing and undulating with vitality. Nearly asleep, we stumble through life, bouncing off expectations, assumptions, and delusions. We tend to accept these externally imposed belief structures as our own. We accept it all as truth, the right way, and build a value structure that chokes out creativity and curiosity. This can lead to *avidya* (ignorance) or misconception, further clouding our understanding of ourselves and the world around us.

When we dare to question these norms, we might feel a bit out of sorts, like we're swimming upstream, out of step with a society that is mostly asleep. To step out of the matrix and follow the call of the heart can feel like you're all alone.

Isolation can be a common experience in this journey of awakening and self-discovery.

The story of Krishna begins with the power of love between Devaki and Vasudeva, a love that shines brightly even in the darkness of their imprisonment. It's this love from which springs the divine creation, Krishna. In the face of greed, fear, despair, and control that Kansa and his minions exhibit, Devaki and Vasudeva bring forth love, beauty, delight, and passion into the world: the avatar of Vishnu in the form of Krishna.

Kansa's tactics of fear, manipulation, and control express the human urge to avoid the inevitable reality of mortality by trying to get, have, own, and consume as much as possible. As Kansa kills all the beautiful, innocent lives of many children to ensure he survives, he tries to outwit his karma. Karma cannot be outwitted, and this we must learn, again and again. No matter what we do to stave off facing our inner demons, our mortality, and avoid projecting them outward, we must eventually face our karma. Kansa's attempt to evade the inevitable backfires, as he is inescapably consumed by Krishna.

We witness the steadfastness of Devaki and Vasudeva even as they are persecuted by the profane—the greedy and desperate attempt to kill love, passion, and goodness. Through Kansa we can see the power of the ego's need to assert itself. We witness how the ego seeks to annihilate anything that might challenge it, even going so far as murdering innocence, imprisoning love, and making desperate attempts to control everything and everyone.

This is evident in every corner of our modern society too, though not so overtly. From the way we treat our living planet, gobbling up every last drop of its resources in an attempt to secure some comfort or position, to the way we treat each other, almost like pawns in our own game of life. It is evident in the way we run our countries, our cities, and also in the way we as individuals attempt to avoid our own deep awakening. We get on the hamster wheel, trying to fulfill an insatiable desire for significance, often getting lost in the matrix, squashing our passions, our love, our tender dance with our hearts, and our deepest longing to feel whole. We find ourselves in servitude to an unending hunger for validation, losing ourselves in the process and distancing ourselves from the divine dance of life, the *rasa lila* that Krishna invites us to join.

When the loving king and queen sneak baby Krishna out and away from certain death, this represents the disruption of the grasping loop of ego-driven desire and control. The imagery of him floating to a small, humble, safe village where he would be raised by loving parents is the triumph of love. We don't even get time to lament his siblings who couldn't make it. We don't have time to grieve the imprisonment of his parents, or even time to celebrate the powerful force of love that allows them to fulfill their dharma and birth a son—a god who would eventually challenge and triumph over the evil, deluded force that is Kansa, the incarnate of shadow force, of the *rakshasa* (demons).

Krishna's childhood in the cowherder village is almost comical in the sense that he, a divine being, is living among ordinary mortals. He's a terrible misfit, yet everyone around him sees him as one of them. This speaks to the tendency of our busy human experience to overlook the divine that dwells within us and among us. It's as if we are sleepwalking, so preoccupied with our daily life that we become blind. We are always searching in other places rather than looking to the simple, the mundane, to discover this remarkable power of love. It's right there among the cow dung of life, in the fertile ground of our everyday experiences. It's only when Krishna eats massive quantities of butter and dirt that he gets caught, and in this moment reveals to his adoptive mother his infinite nature and the nature that is in all things.

We then see the *gopis* in their mundane everyday lives with their responsibilities, living in the fabric of a society constructed before they arrived. But when they hear the enchanting melody of Krishna's flute, it evokes the call of life from within, a call they can no longer ignore. This call is a reflection on those moments when we buck the norm, the unspoken expectations, and follow the call of our deeper longing.

The way each one of the *gopis* leaves their station in life seems abrupt and almost erratic, but what we don't see here is how long that call has been tamped down for, how many times it's been ignored. From dropping dishes to kicking over the milk bucket, we behold this moment of remembering for the *gopis*, an inner transformation as they heed the call of their hearts.

The journey they individually take toward the center of the circle requires them to walk through the darkness and confusion of the forest, unable to see the horizon or a clear direction. They must listen carefully to be guided through the shadow of the forest trees to make their way toward the powerful call. This image brings to light the process, the introspective journey we must take when we question the path we're on and whether it's in service to our deepest calling. When we begin to listen to that inner call, it often feels like this; we can't ignore it, we must go toward it, but we have no clue where we're headed. Like the *gopis* walking through the dark and crowded forest, we too must pay close attention along the way to make sure we are indeed moving in the direction of this call.

When the *gopis* finally emerge from the forest to find Krishna waiting for them in the clearing, they experience a profound sense of relief and exhilaration. Similarly, in our own lives this moment of clarity can happen in meditation, in nature, in an interaction, in movement—in anything we undertake that requires trust in something we can't see. It's the moment when the uncertainty clears and we become crystal clear that our efforts have brought us into this clearing to dance with life, with the divine.

The concept that each *gopi* sees her own individual Krishna and doesn't perceive the others brings to light our personal relationship with our individual connection to the source of light within us all. It also expresses the fact that life is always waiting for us to set aside our fears, our endless stories, and our projections into future and past, and instead fully immerse ourselves in the present, to be right here with life, to open our arms and dance with what is right in front of us.

As the dance begins, the process of full presence takes over. Past and future, good and bad, right and wrong—all dualities drop away. We become lost in the swirl of presence as we spin, celebrate, and awaken to the natural rhythm within us, the beat of our heart and the sacred song deep in our being.

The *gopis* giving their hand to Krishna symbolizes our own commitment to the bond with our own heart when we finally turn our mind toward our center. The moment that happens we are transported into cadence, into an expression of bhakti, and the stuff of *doing* dissolves and the power of *being* takes over.

As the dance grows and the fervor elevates, we experience moments of liberation, of being relieved of the constant thinking, calculating, managing, and manipulating. We let go, giving ourselves freely to the rhythms of the dance, lost in its power to drop us into the now of the moment, where we own nothing except the breath.

With perfect unison, we pound out the beat through the feet, as the earth reverberates its billions of years of evolution up and through us. Dance. Dance. Dance. We are lost and found in this ancient dance, swirling, whirling, rising, and falling. We are in *samavesha*, complete immersion in the divine moment.

When we think of a divine moment, we often think it has to be a mountaintop moment, but it doesn't. The divine moment is in the dance with conflict, frustration, confusion, love, hate, getting what we want, and not getting what we want. It's divine because it's here and now, and we're living it; we are alive and fully participating.

Krishna is associated with the path of bhakti, the yoga of the heart, the path of love; and one of bhakti's translations is "participation." This goes back to the early social movements of direct access to the divine, of participation with others to call in the divine. Bhakti allowed for an intimate and personal connection with God, a direct line to the source, and a path back to wholeness through devotion.

Bhakti's path of devotion emphasizes wholeness. We must include all of ourselves to become whole. It is the opposite of restraining and pushing away parts of oneself to arrive at some illusory perfection, the opposite of some notion of purity devoid of our humanness that cuts us off from Krishna, from vitality, from passion, from life. When we engage with life, we must include all of it and all of ourselves and all of life, even the parts we don't like.

Bhakti evolved over time, and somewhere along the path the practices and mantras escaped the sacred temples and began to circulate among a wider audience through the power of chanting. With chanting, more and more people came running toward the heart of *kirtan* (call-and-response mantra), and remembered their divinity.

Today we can all engage with this connection to God. We can all drop our busy doing self and run toward the heart and dance with our personal Krishna.

It is a reflection of our nature that at the apex of this dance we witness our natural urge to hold on tightly. This expresses our desire to own, have, control, and manipulate this free and limitless commodity of love. Our attempts to label and grasp something that is ungraspable makes the very thing we're trying to keep and hold on to disappear. This grasping creates so much suffering.

Look at social media. We often have an experience and want to hold on to it, use it for validation, becoming so stuck in consuming experiences and people that we miss the magic of simply being present and receiving what is being offered in that moment.

As human beings, we love certainty, and this creates a desire to freeze everything in place, to cling to things in an attempt to preserve them as they are. Recently the entire planet experienced a pandemic that created so much suffering. There was suffering because of loss of life and loss of assumed freedoms, but importantly there was also a loss of what we thought life should be, because it had been that way before.

In the story, Radha exemplifies the beauty of living in the present moment. Keeping her hands soft and open, and simply dancing in the flow of presence, she actually gets the thing she wants most: the love of Krishna. When she opens her eyes and sees Krishna still there, she holds no desire to own, claim, and grasp him, the moment, or the feeling. The *ananda* (bliss) of pure awareness without a desire to freeze it—this state of *being*—is her complete liberation.

We can also find our complete liberation if we learn to simply love, experience, and dance with whatever is happening, acknowledging the transience of it all, with soft eyes and open palms, knowing that all things come and go, rise and fall, begin and end and begin again. The dance of life is forever happening; we simply need to join it and allow it to take us into the grace of our heart. The *hridayam* (heart) is the home of deep devotion to love. We learn to join the dance of this heart even in the mundane, the routine, the responsibilities of life. But it's tricky, for can we be in our daily lives and still dance with the heart? Can we engage in the mundane and still listen for the call of Krishna's flute?

The story of *rasa lila* is a warning about a life of grasping. Trying to name, hold down, and own this infinite, endless connection to the source will only leave us empty-handed and tightfisted. Instead, it is the willingness to hold it all lightly, with open palms, that allows for the connection to the great dance of life. It allows us to stay connected deeply to our heart center without trying to attach ourselves to outer pleasures to fix or solve our discomforts or fill our inner voids.

We are all a part of the divine play, interconnected and impermanent. Not one of us is separate, and each one of us arrives in a body and is guaranteed to depart from that body. During our brief time here we have the chance to run to the heart's clearing and to open our palms and dance wildly, freely, without regard for earlier or later. When we do this, we are truly free and immersed in the moment. This is *samavesha*, the complete immersion into the present.

The gift and preciousness of this life can be easily missed. We're here for a blip, each one of us an expression of the divine essence, yet we often get lost in our personal narratives, cravings, and aversions, losing sight of the dance that is ever-present.

So let us remember, let us run to the heart of life and bathe ourselves in the dance with palms open and soft as rose petals. I will meet you there.

Hare Krishna, Krishna Krishna!

MYTH INTO PRACTICE: EMBRACING THE PLAY OF LIFE

Mantra

Hare Krishna, hare Krishna.
Krishna Krishna, hare hare.
Hare Ram, hare Ram.
Ram Ram, hare hare.
I dance freely through the play of life.
Sri radhe, radhe Govinda.
Sri radhe, radhe Gopal.

Meditation

Sit with your spine tall and face soft. Rest the back of your hands on your legs with the palms open to the sky. As you close your eyes, soften the palms of your hands. With the eyes closed, bring your attention to your inner ears, and begin listening to the breath arriving and departing. As you relax into this rhythm of breath, begin listening more deeply for the call of the heart within you. Listen for the song of compassion and love that lives at your center. Allow yourself to awaken to the song of your heart. As you return to the doing world, bring with you this song.

Movement

Standing or seated, begin swaying your body, becoming quiet and listening to the inward call. Moving from the mechanical nature of tasks to a sway or a circular movement allows us to connect to an inner flow and deep inward listening.

After a few minutes of slow movement, start picking up the rhythm. You can move at any pace—fast, slow, or in between. If you are called to do so, you can stand up to move your feet and your arms. Twirl in circles, kick your legs, and sweep your arms through space in wide, joyful motions. Feel whatever rhythm (music, breath, heartbeat) moves through you.

Eventually start to slow the movements. As the breath settles into a natural rhythm, place both hands, one on top of the other, over your heart. Allow your open palms to sink in toward the rhythm of your heartbeat. Settle into a seated position, rotating the spine in a spiral motion while paying attention to the energy in and around the entire spinal column.

Exercises

1. Set time aside for nine days specifically to dance. It doesn't matter what it looks like, how long it lasts, or whether you've got music; just stop what you're doing and move. Dance as often as possible, even if it's just in your office chair or swaying a little. Meet the dance of life with open palms and a willingness to flow with it.

2. Play some of your favorite music, and sit down with pen and paper to write down what you can hear your heart calling for.

3. Take time to observe life with a sense of wonder and play. Play meaning "fun," but also as in a theater play. Start paying attention to our many characters, and instead of being owned by any of them or being lost within any particular character, pull back and see that it's an ever-evolving dance.

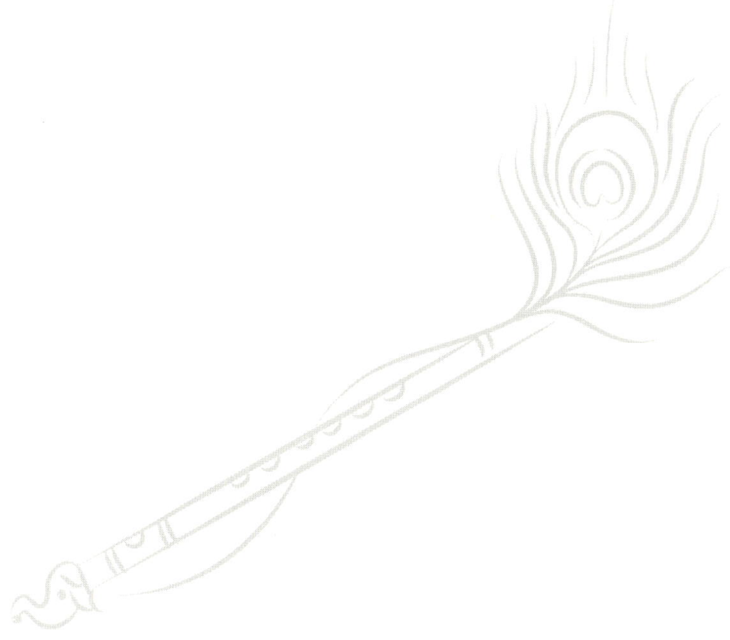

Shiva and Shakti— Descending Ascending

In the boundless span of time, a timeless era with no beginning and no ending, there existed a union so rich and complete that none ever matched it before or since. The home of Shiva and Shakti was a vast spaciousness of infinite openness. Shiva, the ever-present energy of creation and destruction, sat in deep meditation, contemplating all of existence and its cycles of coming and going, dreaming up the finite within the infinite. His body, strong and upright, rippled with muscles showing his strength, but he exuded calm, endless expansiveness. Shakti, the embodiment of pure energy, expression, desire, and movement, languished in her boredom. Her eyes were piercing and alert, and her lithe body was ready for an adventure.

While Shiva sat in repose for thousands of years, Shakti bore her loneliness and had run out of ways to entertain herself. Her deepest and purest desire was to express herself to the world in dynamic and inspired ways. She longed for Shiva to awaken from his meditative state and rejoin her to act out the great dance of love, life, children, and union in a creative flow of form and formlessness. However, he didn't budge from his deep trance. With two of his eyes closed and his third eye open, he sat in utter stillness while her restlessness grew, driving her to new delirium.

With built-up grievances and utter frustration, one day Shakti decided to draw Shiva's attention through a playful game. She came up behind him, placed her hands on his closed eyes, and whispered, "Guess who?" There was no response, only silence. She removed her hands and stomped around in a fit of resentment, only to come back with new resolve. In a fateful fit of impulse, this time she decided to cover Shiva's third eye.

Excitement and anticipation bubbled within Shakti as she waited for Shiva to respond. It felt to her like forever, like time had stopped, as she became overwhelmed by doubt. But the thought of her beloved returning to her arms to create together as they'd done for millennia filled her with joy and readiness, her body charged with an electric energy. She felt sure he was about to stir, and her visceral response was elation.

But instead, a rumbling began, softly at first, then growing into a divine awakening within her. Shakti felt a pulsating surge, like *shaktipat*, the full force of all the universe's energy, inside her. The rumbling intensified, shaking the very fabric of time and space. It dislodged her from her position behind Shiva, moving her directly in front of him. Shiva's awakening form before her revealed his twisted brow, pinched face, and lips turned down in burgeoning rage. Shakti's own face was a mass of confusion, her anticipation reaching fever pitch as panic suddenly washed over her.

Around them, clouds began to form and stir. Roiling in ominous patterns, they rushed around the couple as the sky turned black and the wind whistled. Soon they were in the center of a tornado of fury. Shakti reached out, shaking Shiva, pleading for him to see her. His third eye slammed shut as his two other eyes opened. But instead of seeing his beloved, all he saw was the darkness of his ferocity. Straddling two worlds, he was overtaken by a flurry of tempestuousness.

Shakti had witnessed her Shiva in every state of being, but never before had she seen such fury directed toward her. Despite her fear, she steadied herself and opened her arms, prepared to receive whatever her beloved had to express. As she closed her eyes and opened her infinite heart, she suddenly felt the ground give way below her. Reaching out she tried to grasp him, but his face slipped through her fingers. In desperation she reached for anything she could, her left hand catching the tail end of the tiger skin he wore. As the storm raged around her, she looked up to see the feet of her beloved, but he seemed oblivious to her plight. She tried to scream, to call out to him, but no sound left her. Her Shiva was unreachable. Tears streamed down her face as she felt her grip on the tiger skin slipping, and she plummeted farther from his sight.

She had wanted to be closer, more connected to her divine love, but all she saw was him fading in the distance. Arms flailing at the nothingness, legs kicking in some nonsensical attempt to get back to her disappearing Shiva, she continued to fall into the void of nothingness until he was completely out of sight.

Shakti's mind felt foggy. She couldn't tell up from down, as she was suspended in pure nothingness. All sensation was gone. She felt nothing; no sadness, no hopes, no love, no loss. There was no before or after, no memory or thought—just an endless, directionless void of unmanifest space. She was suspended for what felt like an eternity, though it was difficult for her to even comprehend the concept of time.

And then without warning Shakti felt a soft caress from below, igniting her senses. Goose bumps spread across her skin as the vague sense of floating for an eternity turned into a distinct sense of falling. An acute awareness of movement enveloped her, her hair blowing upward as if she were descending rapidly through the air. Her lungs filled and emptied rhythmically. She felt a true sense of descending through space, enveloped by cool, fresh air.

As the seemingly endless fall continued, she noticed tiny particles whizzing past her, creating friction that brought a newfound sensation: warmth. The heat enveloped her skin, accompanied by a radiant glow from within and without, infusing her with reinvigorating energy and crystal clarity.

Then the luminous glow began to feel softer and softer, melting into her body as a watery warmth washed over her. She became aware of the saliva in her mouth, the pulse of blood through her veins, and a sense of pouring through the sky. She continued to cascade downward until finally her body met a hard, solid surface.

Thud. The ground. Terra firma.

She lay there for a long time, feeling gravity pushing her down onto this hard surface, absorbing the unfamiliar sensation and smell. The solidity was both startling and comforting, a grounding contrast to the unending void she had just traversed.

Earth. Having never experienced dirt, earth, so solid, so tangible, Shakti's senses were alive with curiosity. She ran her hands across the earth, her fingernails plowing through the dirt, each grain and pebble a universe of new sensation. She grabbed handfuls of soil, inhaling its potent strength, rolling over to bury her body in it, delighting in each grain against her skin.

As she connected physically with the earth, her body discovered its new firmness, her bones and flesh responding to the constraints of gravity in an intoxicating embrace. She stood up, feeling the earth communicate through her feet, the energy rising through her, bringing stability up her spine. The earth and her own form didn't feel separate; the ground spoke to her and her body spoke to the ground.

Bolstered by this deep connection, Shakti began to explore the new world around her—every crevice, nook, fold, valley, mountain, and forest. Her hands and her feet traced the solid contour of the earth, dug into the base of trees, and traced their roots. Lying on the forest floor, she absorbed the whispers of fungi, molds, earthworms, and the billions of years of evolution pulsing through her body, remembering the ancient wisdom of the universe held in each grain of dirt.

But after thousands of years of this solid exploration, Shakti began to feel heavy and stuck. A whisper called to her. A silent something nudged at her. Was it Shiva? She wouldn't know, for she had no memory of him.

The once exhilarating solidity now felt limiting, binding Shakti in unexpected ways. She wandered about until she came across a tiny trickling stream. The sound of the water called to her, drawing her to splash and slurp and immerse her toes in the cool, flowing current. It was a relief, a balm to her weary spirit, and precisely what she didn't know she was searching for, what she deeply needed. As she followed the course of the stream, she was mesmerized by the smooth liquid swirling around her, hardly noticing as it widened and deepened, enveloping her completely.

Shakti floated in the river, which transformed into a vast delta, her envelopment dissolving as she became one with the water. Goose bumps rippled across her skin as she surrendered to the current that guided her to the river's mouth, opening wide to the endless ocean. The water turned salty and tumultuous, swelling to the shore and retreating back, its endless movements filling her with pure awe.

Riding the ocean's swells, calm one moment and wildly undulating the next, she found herself riding the peaks and valleys with no preference for one over the other. Ascending to a wave crest, she looked across at all of the other crests looking back at her, and the momentary thought of "my peak versus another peak" arose. But in that very instant she remembered that every wave, every peak, emerged from the same vast ocean, from the same source.

The cyclical ebb and flow, the undulating of her body with the tides, and the buildup and release of energy all resonated within her, awakening an ancient understanding. She felt the rhythmic push and pull, echoing the beat of her heart and the rise and fall of her breath.

For thousands of years Shakti floated in the fluid nature of her being, immersed in the ways of water, flowing, diving, and splashing through all things water. But eventually the perpetual dampness seeped into her, leaving her cold, shivering, and bordering on dissolution. The lines between her and the vast waters blurred until she felt she might lose her definition and break apart into a billion droplets. Slowly pulling herself out of the seemingly endless waters and dripping on the shore, she quivered, cold to the marrow.

Still guided by that internal whisper she could not name, Shakti sought warmth to chase away the dampness and chill, rubbing her hands to generate heat. Longing to increase this heat, she rubbed sticks together to create fire. Illuminated by the fire's glow, she embarked on a quest for the essence of fire. This journey took her to volcanoes spewing molten rock, through wildfires ravaging the land, and under the warm rays of the sun caressing her skin. She grew fierier with a distinct clarity, perception, and powerful will to assert herself in the world—making things and burning them down, flashing into bursts of anger, and eventually becoming overwhelmed with the feeling that she was going to burn up from the inside out.

Seeking refuge from this sensation of burning, Shakti climbed the highest mountain, reaching her arms into the cooling breeze. The wind's soothing touch immediately tempered her fiery essence. Her exhalations became longer and softer, and her mind cooled and filled with magical thoughts and visions, goose bumps returning across her skin to enliven her whole body. Air filled her lungs and flowed back out, the exchange between her inner world and the outer becoming her new rhythm of life.

But despite the equilibrium she found in the elements, Shakti eventually felt a deep, inexplicable longing, a yearning she could not shake off. After thousands of years of exploring her connection with the elements, a desire to return to something unnamed began to overtake her every thought.

She meditated, seeking answers and a stillness of mind. In meditation on the mountaintop, she repeatedly envisioned herself reuniting with an unknowable force that balanced her, yet she had no memory of where she'd come from, the divinity she was, the union she'd danced in for eons. A faint whisper of her true origin kept returning, kept tugging at her.

One day Shakti opened her eyes from meditation and began building a mound of dirt, adding water to it and giving it the form of a clay emblem—the linga—thrusting up toward the sky. She sat around it meditating day and night. As she meditated, she felt her consciousness expanding, her being growing lighter, seemingly unbound by gravity. Her whole existence seemed to levitate and ascend.

Not only was she ascending in her awareness, but she could also feel a familiar force descending to meet her. Finally the whisper, the call, the unknown longing was revealed: to return to her beloved Shiva. Flooded with ecstasy, they embraced, holding the balance of the embodiment of earth, form, body, and the infinite and limitlessness bounds of consciousness. Shiva and Shakti reunited, restoring the harmony and divine embrace of the perfect union, from finite to infinite, once again.

MYTH AND MEANING: FORM AND FORMLESSNESS

This purana attempts to reveal to our human minds the concept of something larger than ourselves and our daily existence and concerns. It suggests that we are more than just what we think we are; we are expressions of nature and the five elements—earth, air, fire, water, and ether (space)—that make up our existence, just like all other living things.

Yet we tend to identify ourselves as something separate, independent from these elements, these building blocks for life on earth. When we pay attention to the balance of energy of each of the individual elements and the kinship of all life, polarities like us and them begin to fade, losing their power to divide us.

Beginning in the space of an infinite, vast expanse and witnessing the expression of determined energy to exist and to experience is the summation of the yogic philosophy. The unmanifest moves into manifest and then back again; this is the *spanda* (grand pulsation) of life and death, the process of embodying and shedding the body.

Through the practice of meditation, we enter the expansive space of Shiva, and through our daily living we ground in the aspect of Shakti. Shiva represents the subtle aspects of our life force, the etheric, the context for which life unfolds. Shakti, on the other hand, represents the more tangible elements of air, fire, water, and earth—the expressive aspects. One can't fully exist without the other. The more etheric nature—the being aspect—can remain spacious, but it longs for expression; the doing aspect longs for spaciousness. These energies support each other in a symbiotic pulse that creates balance between doing and being.

What we mostly witness and value, in both ourselves and the world around us, is doing. Society rewards action—the doing part—with awards, accolades, money, and stuff, boosting our ego *ahamkara* (ego) and creating a sense of separation between the self and the rest of the universe. The Shiva part—the simple beingness of life, a breath, a mind, and a body—often gets lost here. This disconnection leads to suffering, as we become subject to the whims of winning and losing, happiness and sadness, birth and death. In forgetting that we are woven from the same fabric as the universe, we inadvertently limit our understanding of our true, divine nature. The drama of daily living makes us forget our connection to something greater, making us miss the exquisiteness of the natural world and the billions of years it's taken for us to be able to be here.

The story opens in the realm of Shiva, as he hovers above the mundane, outside the messiness of embodiment, and instead rests in the endless expanse of time and space. Shakti, at this point, is suspended in Shiva's world, yet she burns for more— for expression, creation, exchange, and energy. Little did she know that her longing to express herself and her energy would take her on such a wild journey, away from Shiva. However, she could no longer repress this need. And so begins her journey.

Shakti's journey is analogous to our own journeys as human beings, landing in physical bodies and arriving in the reality of energy embodied as form. This arrival, this journey into embodiment, comes with awkwardness, helplessness, discovery, wonder, pain, discomfort, learning, gravity, and most of all a forgetting of our divine interconnectedness with all beings across all space and time. Instead, for the time we're here we become solidly self-centered, adopting the I/me/mine mentality, losing track of the power of the life force that is breathed into us. The fall of Shakti represents our descent into the experience of four of the elements and into *maya*, the illusion of separation.

First we witness Shakti's relationship with earth as she lands on the solid ground. We see her coat her body with dirt and mud, and smell the rich scents of the soil, grounding herself in her surroundings. Immersed in her discovery of earth, Shakti also finds her own earthly essence through the hardness of her bones, the strength of her teeth and the firmness of her muscles. Earth is the densest expression of prana (life force), and due to gravity, the body evolved to be dense and solid. There is power in being barefoot on earth; direct contact with the earth boosts our natural immune system more effectively than any vitamin or medicine. Our connection to the earth helps us rest our busy brains and truly appreciate the strength of what's below our feet.

Shakti then encounters a trickling stream and becomes enthralled with this new fluid, mysterious, and persistent element. She experiences water's refreshing and elusive nature as it pours through her hands and drips off her body. She laps at it and drinks it, holding it in her mouth, swishing it around and exploring the taste with the sense organ of water, the tongue.

Water is cohesion, the circulatory lifeblood of our biological systems. With 55 to 60 percent of the human body made of water, the entirety of it is pulsing with the flow of water. So when Shakti immerses herself in the expanding river, she is in a sense immersing herself into her body's most natural state, a state of coherence.

Through her immersive exploration, we witness the ebb and flow, the undulations of life and emotions, and the immense capacity for water to move mountains. This shape-shifting element can wear through the densest of boulders and carve vast valleys. In Shakti's discovery of water, we have an opportunity to glimpse the power of our own inner fluidity and the need to create flow when we get stuck. The tidal motion of our emotions is a prime example of the power of water to help us wash away the boulder-sized blockage of big emotions. When stuck in hardened patterns, fluidity can break us free. This transformation, from a solid state of being stuck to a liquid fluidity, is where we find some of the most potent solutions. While melting the glacier of our old stuck behaviors and addictions is not easy, and sometimes it might feel easier to stay frozen, we witness Shakti bravely give herself over to the flow.

However, too much immersion in water, being so fluid that we become boundaryless, can also get us into trouble. We may move through the world not knowing where someone ends and we begin, confusing their emotions with our own, and pouring ourselves into everything and everyone. This boundarylessness can cause us to neglect our own body, mind, and spirit. It shows up when we can't say a clear no at the cost of our own well-being. When we feel resentful or overwhelmed, it's vital to check in and see how we got there. Often it's because we lack boundaries and are unable to speak up and protect our own precious life resources.

To escape the perpetual dampness of water, Shakti discovers heat and fire. As she sits, sings, and dances around the fire, the heavy, saturated feeling of water begins to burn off, revealing her deeper wisdom. The embers floating past her eyes help her realize that her sight and perception have come into greater focus. Sight is the sense organ of fire, of seeing clearly without misperceptions. Fire offers discernment and can burn through our delusions—fantasies based on old conditioning, traumas, and experiences. Fire has the power to blaze through these and reveal reality.

A large proportion of yoga (and Ayurveda) practices are predicated on tending to the fire as a way to transmute karmas (cause and effect) and lead the way toward clear perception. When Shakti explores fire, we get a glimpse at our own potential to transmute old beliefs and stagnant patterns. The vibrancy that comes with a consistent tending of our own inner flame is called *tejas*, the radiance of disciplined practice that radiates into all areas of our lives, bringing healing, integration, and experiences of wholeness to our entire being.

Just like a forest fire can clear out the old and dead, creating space to birth new life, when we work through old ways of reacting and allow a new perspective, we create new pathways and new inner growth. However, fire, although a potent instrument for healing, also holds equal power of destruction. Out of balance, fire can manifest as anger, aggression, inflammation, absolutes, and burning out of control. This is the dance with fire: It can warm, illuminate, cook, distill, and discern, or it can destroy.

When Shakti feels the fire burn too deeply, she wanders to the mountaintop to catch the wind and cool the raging fire. With a rush of fresh air in her lungs, she feels intertwined with all other breathing creatures as their exhalation becomes her inhalation and vice versa. The air awakens her creative thinking, prompting her to move freely on the mountaintop, awash in the breeze.

Air is the element of lightness, motion, breath, and oxygen. It fosters the flow of thought and movement. It's the element that connects us to all living things by facilitating exchange between our internal and external worlds. Our exhalation brings our internal world outward, where it joins the collective, and our inhalation brings the collective into us. This interconnectedness became more apparent during the pandemic. On an energetic level, we can notice how the breath, energy, and life force of all living things nearby affect us. When we pay attention to the interconnectedness of this very breath we share with trees, oceans, root and fungi systems, soil, atmosphere, animals, and each other, we wake up and desire to care for this precious ecosystem.

The *rishis* (sages) associated air with prana, or life force, as our life energy is carried on the breath. Shakti's interest in mastering the breath offers insight into the teachings of pranayama, the practice of guiding and controlling our breath, which is an integral part of yoga. Through pranayama we can directly stimulate or calm our vagal nervous system, boosting our immune system so that we can regenerate, heal, digest, and return to vitality.

Through her explorations with earth, water, fire, and air, we see a longing welling up in Shakti's heart, a call for something more intangible, incalculable, etheric. This unknowable, untouchable, unnameable force grips her heart, arousing a sense of wonder, longing, and thirst to unite with this elusive essence.

Beyond the tangible aspects of earth, water, fire, and air is the etheric element, or *aakasha*, the element associated with the unseen and subtle forces that connect all of existence. It is closely linked to vibrations and sound, which are fundamental to creation and perception. Shabda is the *tanmatra* (subtle essence) of the ether, representing the primal sound and vibrations that permeate the universe.

In our own lives we can connect with this etheric element when we quiet our minds and become mindful, when we slow down enough to feel the spaces within our windpipe, in our nasal passages, within our ears, and eventually between our thoughts and actions. These moments of stillness can allow us to feel the vibrations and subtle energies that are always present but go unnoticed in our busy lives. By tuning into these vibrations, we can tap into the etheric element and experience a deeper connection to the universe and all of existence.

Shakti's longing overwhelms her, and we witness her build a linga to bring her higher and closer to the expanse of the ether. She meditates, sitting with the stillness of her mind until she eventually reunites with her beloved Shiva, and in that moment a flood of remembering washes over her, a profound revelation that they were never truly separated; it only *felt* that way.

This union of Shiva and Shakti reflects the concept of *samavesha,* complete immersion with the divine. It's the feeling of oneness with everything that is, all that ever was, and all that will be—the lack of separation and the sense of unity that underlines our very existence. This profound realization and experience can serve as a reminder of the interconnectedness and the essence of all life. By choosing to wake out of the stupor of small dramas and the confines of old narratives, we can potentially recognize the grandeur of existence. Spending even a few moments of our life in this recognition can fill us with a sense of utter wonder and greater appreciation.

Shakti's journey, touching all life with wonder and awe until she longs for the ultimate reconnection with Shiva, is the expression of the path of yoga. It's a path of seeing and experiencing divinity in all things. It's a journey that invites us to remember, reconnect, and realign ourselves with all of the elements, tangible and intangible, fostering a sense of unity and interconnectedness that underscores the essence of our existence.

MYTH INTO PRACTICE: BALANCE

Mantra

Om hrim shivaya namaha.

I bow to the pure infinite creative energy, Shakti (*hrim*), and the pure undifferentiated consciousness (Shiva).

Or:

I am finite and infinite.

Meditation

Sit comfortably and connect with your breath. Bring your attention to the earth element within the body. Invite yourself to dive into a sense of wonder about the world around us. Consider the billions of years of evolution, life, and decay, that created everything around you—the dirt, invisible microbes, the flowers and the insects that pollinate them, the technology that allows us to live in such comfort, the stars and galaxies beyond our comprehension—whatever comes to mind. Invite yourself to sit in awe of what is around you and within you. Scan your own body and consider the universe of cells and fluids and systems within that animate and sustain it.

Movement

Finding a place in nature where you feel comfortable, remove your shoes and step onto the earth, grass, or sand. Closing your eyes, wiggle your toes and feel the ground below your feet and feel for the elements of earth, water, fire, air, and space around you and within you. Opening your eyes, begin to walk slowly with attention on every footfall and the sensation of your feet on the earth. Eventually come to a stop, reach your arms out wide, then overhead. Then place them together and draw the hands in prayer to your heart. Now repeat this, once for each element.

Exercises

1. Pay attention to the natural world and look for the relationship between yourself and the elements.

2. Write down which element you most relate to and how it shows up in your life. Then write how you relate to the Shiva and Shakti energy in your daily life.

IN THE END

In the midst of the third trimester of my second full-term pregnancy, I found myself grappling with what I can only describe as depression. I had lost my way to hope, resilience, and my usual I-can-do-anything mindset. Instead, an ooze of negative thoughts and feelings clogged my mind and body. At a time when I expected to be filled with excitement and anticipation, tempered perhaps by a little realistic fear (once you give birth, you forever know what it takes to move a life into the world), I instead felt overwhelmed by a nearly suffocating weight of grief and despair. I felt I had nothing to offer and was riddled with guilt for bringing a new life into this nothingness. Despite trying all of my practices, following all of the advice, and continuing to teach and practice yoga, I couldn't escape this emotional sinkhole.

Like my first birth, I had chosen to labor and birth at home, and the day had arrived. My water broke the day before, so the pressure for her arrival was on. Desperate for sleep that eluded me, I spent the first part of the night in bed, wandering the hallways of my mind until I decided to get up and wander the hallways of our home instead. Pacing. I felt the pain growing. Pacing. I felt the weight of the gloom as I moved with an intensity back and forth, from the kitchen sink to the living room window. Back and forth.

At 4:30 in the morning, with darkness still enveloping the outside, an extraordinary quiet fell upon our home. My husband and daughter slept in the room below. The internal noise and the creaking of the floorboards quieted, and I paused at the window to watch the shadowy dance of a tree in the moonlight. From somewhere far beyond I heard whispers, faint at first, but growing louder by the minute: *Everything is going to be okay. You have everything you need to get through this. You've got this . . .* In that moment I felt like Hanuman as he climbed the mountain alone to go inward and meditate. He had hit the edge of the world, his limit, and had no solution in sight. However, when he opened his eyes he was surrounded by his community reminding him of his superpowers, reminding him that he could fly.

You've got this. I could hear my community, my family, my ancestors' voices reminding me of my superpowers. *You've got this.* Whatever darkness was pulling me down lifted, and a flame of power and grace washed over me. In that moment I felt the strength of Hanuman when he gets ready to leap alone across the ocean and into the fire.

Feeling empowered as the pain grew sharp and piercing and the downward pressure nearly unbearable, the feeling of being alone faded as I felt my baby, ancestors, and community all gathered around me. The vision of Hanuman realizing he could fly played through my mind as my beloved child arrived into this world.

This lived experience of profound personal revelation during my labor resonated deeply with the timeless truths found in the puranas. These ancient texts, with their deep reservoirs of wisdom, are woven through the tapestry of my entire life, reminding me of the human condition, bringing light when I get lost in the dark, and exposing nuance and complexity when I get stuck in a small point of view. They offer me hope and compassion as I move through the great play of life, guiding me through its tumultuous scenes with the steadiness of inherited wisdom.

This experience emphasizes how even though the puranas are from a different time that is hard to relate to, they allow us to travel into realms unseen and touch the fabric of the human condition and the human experience of the collective consciousness. By experiencing the stories through the characters of another era, we can absorb their essence, their wisdom, and their teachings, helping us connect to our present world. In today's hyperconnected world stories are more potent than ever. They traverse digital landscapes, breaking barriers and forging global connections. I could be sitting five thousand miles away from the place where these stories originate, and yet I can hear them, draw meaning from them, live them, and experience them. They are dynamic, told in thousands of different versions across different contexts and in different voices. They are simply meant to be that way: changeable, adaptable, and moldable to awaken new perspectives, to shine a light on our blind spots, to help us understand our universe.

These ancient tales enable us to step back from our established perspectives, our very subjective preconceptions and frameworks, and see the world through a wider lens. As we read or listen to one ancient purana after another, we notice their power to help us break stereotypes and transcend societal norms and expectations. In stories we find the profound truth that in every ending lies a new beginning, and in every beginning the echoes of tales long told. They remind us of who we are, where we come from, and where we are headed. So thank you for playing this game of telephone with me, and coming along with my sharing of these ancient tales that have awakened me.

In sharing these ancient tales, we've journeyed through the annals of mythology right into our souls, for within every tale, every character, and every twist, there lies a fragment of us, a shard of our own story. In their depths we discover the myriad faces of our being. The hero, the villain, the sage, the teacher—each character is a reflection of our own desires, dilemmas, and dreams. Through them we traverse the labyrinth of our own psyche, seeking answers, finding questions, and unveiling and understanding the mystery of our own existence.

As we draw to a close on this tapestry of tales, let us remember that in the echoing chambers of history, where countless tales have been told and retold, it's our own unique journey, our own myth that holds the deepest resonance. Every soul is a universe of stories waiting to be unveiled. As we journey through the pages of life, remember that to truly live is to craft our own tale, to embrace the unknown, and to unfold the myth that is uniquely ours, the story that unlocks the mysteries of our universe and the timeless dance of our existence.

These are *your* stories now!

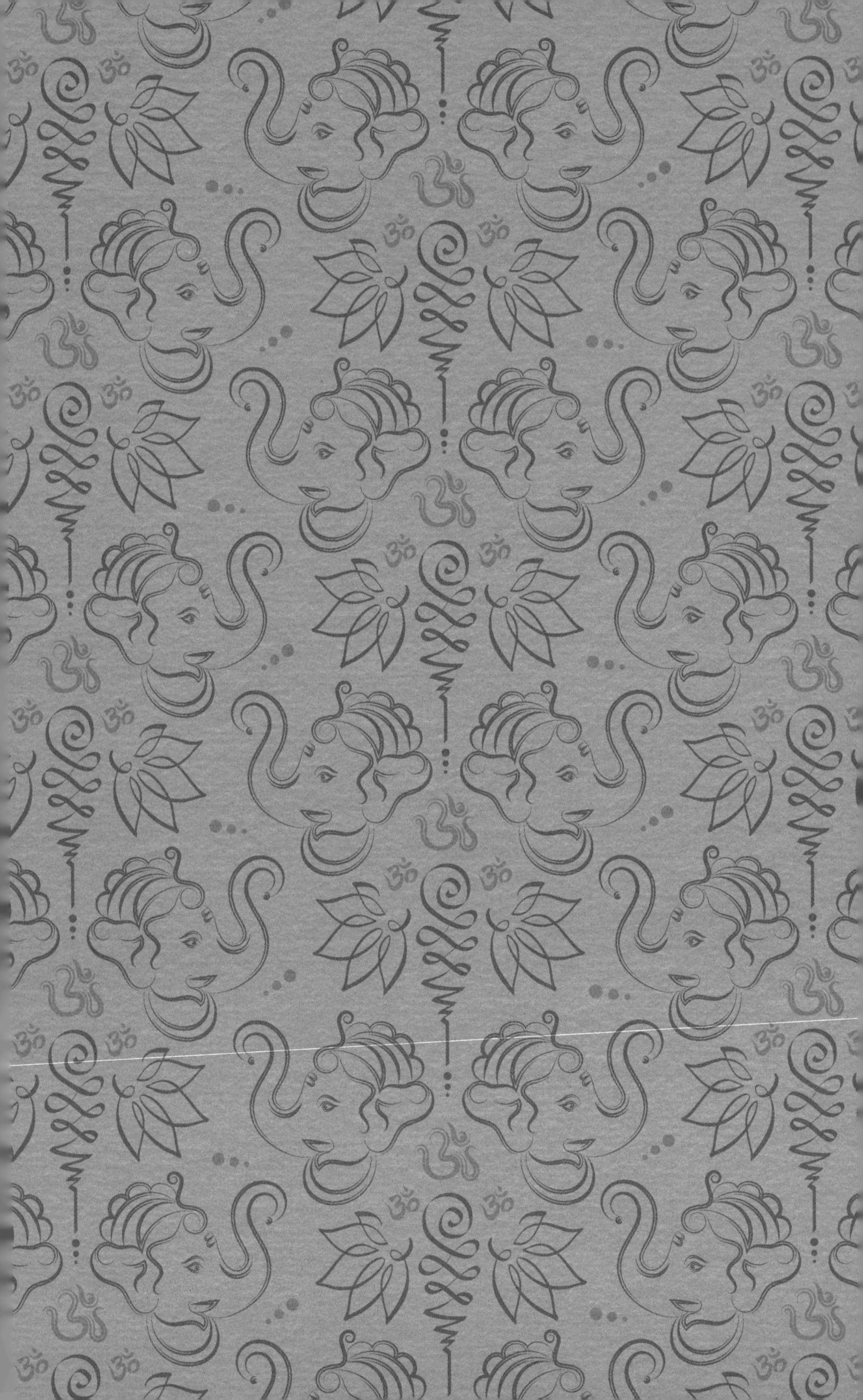

ACKNOWLEDGMENTS

To my children, India and Lilianna. These stories were once your lullabies, carrying you into sleep, and now you are carrying them forward in the way you live, love, and create. You remind me daily that the heart of mythology is not in the telling alone, but in the living. May the stories you write with your lives continue to ripple outward, linking us across time and lineage.

I owe a profound debt of gratitude to Vinitha Agarwal, Connie Engel, and Lauren Shufran, whose invaluable contributions shaped the essence and depth of these pages. Your insights were transformative, and these words carry your wisdom and dedication within them.

With heartfelt appreciation to Raoul Goff, Phillip Jones, and Tania Casselle for your unwavering belief and encouragement that fueled this endeavor.

The voices of my paternal grandmother, grandfather, great-grandmother, father, mother, and sister echo in my ear as these stories unfold.

To Hareesh Wallis, Jody Greene, Max Strom, Adyashanti, Prem Rawat, and Shiva Kumar—thank you for touching my heart, guiding my path, and reminding me of the spaciousness within story and silence alike. To all the teachers and storytellers whose narratives have illuminated and enriched my understanding of life, I bow in gratitude.

And finally, to the flow of voices that have kept these tales alive through endless retelling, creating an unbroken chain of meaning across time—thank you. And to the listeners whose presence, commitment, and curiosity encouraged this book into being and gave these stories renewed vitality and relevance.

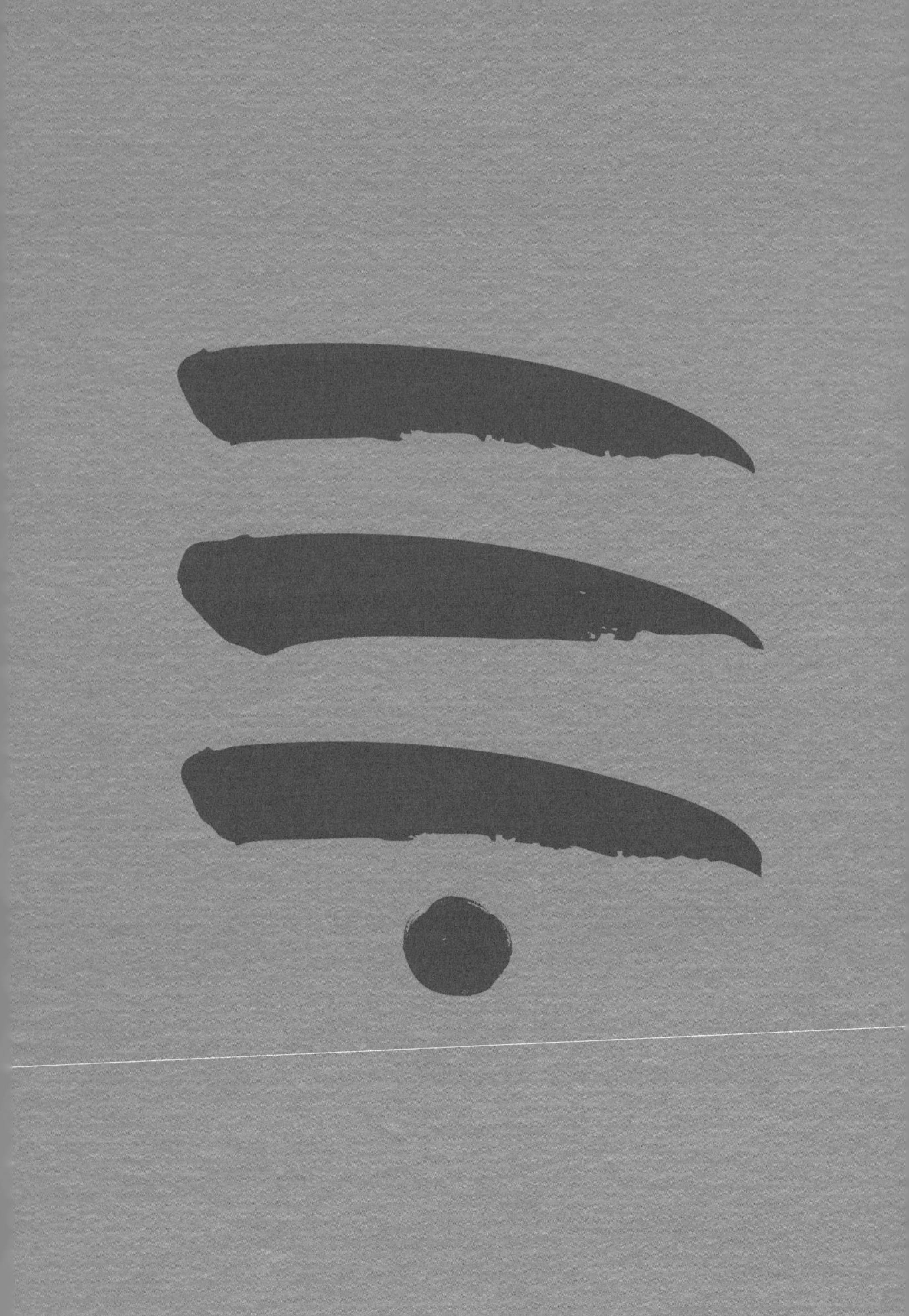

ABOUT THE AUTHOR

Janet Stone's yoga journey began at seventeen under Maharaji, her meditation teacher, whose reverence for simplicity and joy live on in her practice and teachings to this day. She shares from the depth of her own sadhana (sustained practice), her studentship in the eight-limbed path, her creative approach to asana, and her reverence for bhakti (devotional, heart-centered yoga, including chanting mantra).

Janet's connection to India through her grandfather, who was born and raised near Hyderabad, along with her own transformative travels to India, infuses her work with reverence for ancient traditions. Drawing from over a dozen years in the film industry, over thirty years of spiritual practice, and twenty-five years of teaching yoga, Janet brings a unique perspective to her writing, blending spiritual insights with a storyteller's heart.

Based in San Francisco, California, Janet continues to share her teachings through classes, retreats, workshops, teacher trainings, devotional albums, and her global online community at JanetStoneYoga.com.